The Source
for
Syndromes 2

Gail J. Richard

Debra Reichert Hoge

Skills: Speech and Language
Ages: Birth through 18

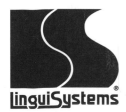

LinguiSystems

LinguiSystems, Inc.
3100 4th Avenue
East Moline, IL 61244-9700

Fax: 800-577-4555
E-Mail: service@linguisystems.c
Web: www.linguisystems.com

800-PRO IDEA
800-776-4332

TDD: 800-933-8331
         (for those with hearing impairments)

ISBN 0-7606-0361-8

D1157529

About the Authors

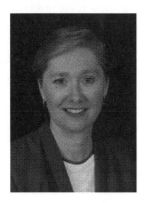

Gail J. Richard, Ph.D., CCC-SLP, is a professor in the Department of Communication Disorders and Sciences at Eastern Illinois University in Charleston. Her responsibilities include undergraduate and graduate courses and clinical diagnostic and therapy supervision. Areas of expertise focus on childhood and adolescent language disorders such as autism, selective mutism, language processing, learning disabilities, and other developmental disorders. Gail's experience prior to joining the university faculty included public school therapy and a diagnostic/therapeutic preschool setting. Gail consults with school districts on a regular basis to problem-solve and assist in educational programming ideas for special needs students. She is a popular presenter for workshops around the country due to the practical nature of the information she shares with her audiences.

Gail's professional honors and awards include Past President and Fellow of the Illinois Speech-Language-Hearing Association, recipient of the Illinois Clinical Achievement Award, Outstanding Alumnus Award at Southern Illinois University-Carbondale, member of the American Speech-Language-Hearing Association's (ASHA's) Legislative Council, five Faculty Excellence Awards, and NCAA Faculty Athletics Representative for Eastern Illinois University. Previous publications with LinguiSystems include *The Source for Syndromes*, *The Source for Autism*, *The Language Processing Test*, and *The Language Processing Kit*, co-authored with Mary Anne Hanner.

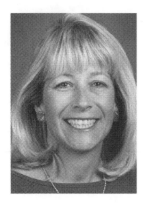

Debra Reichert Hoge, Ed.D., CCC-SLP, is an associate professor in the Department of Special Education and Communication Disorders at Southern Illinois University in Edwardsville. She teaches undergraduate and graduate courses in early intervention, child language development and disorders, low incidence populations, and early childhood special education courses. Prior to becoming a faculty member at Southern Illinois, Debra taught in the public schools and at a center for autism. Debra has presented numerous workshops throughout the country on early intervention; assessment and intervention with infants, toddlers, and their families; and early childhood special education issues. She was chosen as an author and presenter on two national in-service grants awarded to the American Speech-Language-Hearing Association (ASHA): ASHA's Building Blocks and ASHA's Interdisciplinary Preschool Project.

Debra is a native and lifelong resident of St. Louis, Missouri, and lives there with her husband, James, and daughter, Jillian Jean. *The Source for Syndromes 2* is Debra's second publication with LinguiSystems. She also co-authored *The Source for Syndromes*.

Dedication

To the research professionals whose efforts provide the scientific information that practitioners rely on to remediate the unique needs of those with syndrome disabilities.

Table of Contents

Introduction

"Every person is an exception."
Soren Kierkegaard

In January 1999, we published *The Source for Syndromes,* the precursor to the book you are holding. Since its publication, we've heard a variety of comments regarding the first book. Here are some of our favorites:

"This book is just what I needed."

"*The Source for Syndromes* is so easy to read."

"You made the syndromes less intimidating."

"I feel more confident about where to start on some really challenging cases."

"I love *The Source for Syndromes!*" (Sorry, had to include this one.)

We loved hearing the comments, but they were often followed by:

"Does *The Source for Syndromes* include _____?"

"Could you do _____ Syndrome?"

"Do you have any information on _____ Syndrome?"

"When are you going to publish something on _____?"

"Have you ever heard of _____ Syndrome?"

It became apparent that *The Source for Syndromes* filled a need for many practicing speech-language pathologists and adjunct professionals working with young children. It was also quite clear that more of the same was needed.

Despite the availability of the Internet and other electronic sources of information, time demands and information overkill exasperate conscientious professionals trying to find current information on childhood disorders. Medical jargon and detail overload in the name of accountability mask the critical aspects of diagnosis and intervention. Surfing the web doesn't always satisfy the immediate questions of "Where do I start?" and "What are the critical aspects in speech-language/communication development?"

So here is *The Source for Syndromes 2*, a sequel and companion to the first book. This volume discusses over 20 additional syndromes. The purpose is the same as in the first book: to delineate the nature of each syndrome as clearly as possible, and to indicate the primary remediation focus for speech-language pathologists. We are NOT trying to provide a definitive, extensive, medically-exhaustive review of the research on each syndrome. The goal is to help professionals understand the syndrome, focus on pertinent aspects of the syndrome, and generate goals and strategies to initiate intervention with preschool children.

Improved medical diagnostic technology leads to the diagnosis of new syndromes every day. It's impossible to include all the syndromes represented by our clients in this book. So we've tried to include a variety of syndromes that belong to a family of similar syndromes, or have similar symptoms associated with them. Don't get discouraged if the specific syndrome attached to your new case isn't included in *The Source for Syndromes 2*. It's likely that your syndrome will be very similar to another one in this book based on *core symptoms* and *speech-language remediation goals*. For example, many syndromes have characteristics originating from structural anomalies like facial feature formation (e.g., cleft palate, nasal passage deviations, conductive hearing losses). The Syndrome Overview in the back of the book will help you locate similar syndromes based on core characteristics and speech-language remediation goals.

Don't get intimidated or frustrated when faced with yet another new syndrome. Instead, acknowledge that while the medical label may be unique, the small child brought to you for help simply presents some very common characteristics seen in numerous cases. It isn't the medical syndrome that makes him or her unique; the child is already special. As professionals, we're challenged with medically-fragile infants and young children who present a composite profile of deficits. The interaction of deviations can be overwhelming when viewed separately. An integration of services offers a more realistic promise for improvement. It's important to see the common elements in many childhood speech-language disorders.

Each chapter is divided into five sections:

- Syndrome Definition

- Behavioral Characteristics Profile

- Speech-Language Issues

- Intervention Issues

- Summary

As the great philosopher Kierkegaard reminds us, each person is exceptional in his or her own right. Within the education and medical professions, exceptionality seems to have become a bad or dreaded thing. We believe that being exceptional is what life is about, and it should be celebrated! Our responsibility as speech-language pathologists is to meet the needs of each exceptional child and also of his/her parents who come to us with hopes and dreams for improvement. We directly affect each child's potential and quality of life. When we strive to help a child reach a higher level of existence, we enhance our own exceptionality by accepting the challenge. It takes courage to embrace exceptions. We hope this book makes the journey a bit more comfortable!

Gail & Deb

Apert Syndrome

Characteristics

- Feeding and breathing problems
- Developmental delays
- Learning disability/mental retardation
- Cleft palate and dental anomalies
- Conductive hearing loss
- Speech-language delays

- premature fusion of bones in the skull

- webbed, claw-like hands

- large, widely-spaced eyes

- 1/100,000 to 1/160,000 live births

- males and females equally affected

- possible hydrocephalus

Syndrome Definition

Apert syndrome is classified as an acrocephalo-syndactyly syndrome due to the primary features: a premature fusion of the bones in the skull (acrocephalo) and webbing or malformations of the hands and feet (syndactyly).

Apert syndrome is considered a relatively rare condition which occurs in a reported range of 1 in 100,000 to 1 in 160,000 live births. Both males and females are affected equally, and the syndrome can be diagnosed at birth, although the facial features tend to become more striking during the preschool years.

It can be inherited as an autosomal-dominant disorder, but most cases are considered to be mutations on the long arm of chromosome 10. Apert is similar to Crouzon, Pfeiffer, and Carpenter syndromes. These syndromes cause cranial anomalies, but unlike in Apert syndrome, limbs remain normal. There are suggestions that older fathers are more at risk for producing children with these syndromes, but the reports have not been substantiated.

In typical newborns, the bones of the skull separate from each other to assist in passage through the birth canal. After birth, the bones fuse together with a fibrous tissue to accommodate brain growth. But in Apert syndrome, the bones fuse prematurely, resulting in noticeable cranial differences. The shape of the head is the most striking feature, with a high, prominent forehead and marked swelling at midline. The back of the head is flattened. The dysmorphic features can become more severe as the head grows during the preschool years. Surgery may be necessary in the early years to correct the premature fusion of the skull.

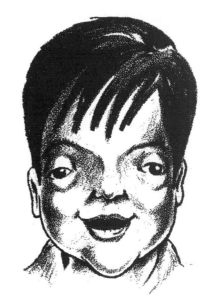

Hydrocephalus can be a complication caused by faulty drainage of fluid in the brain. A hydrocephalic condition might be missed in early stages because of the unusual shape of the skull. If hydrocephalus is present, it will be necessary to insert a shunt to drain excess fluid away from the brain.

Facial features include large prominent eyes which are spaced widely apart. The nose is small and the nasal bridge is flattened, often resulting in breathing and feeding difficulty in the first few months. Ears can be set low on the head and congenital hearing loss occurs frequently due to bilateral malformation of the middle ear space and structures. Approximately 30% of individuals with Apert syndrome present with a cleft of the soft palate and dental abnormalities, including an open bite and crowded teeth.

Limb malformations vary, but webbing between the fingers occurs frequently. The worst cases evidence fusion of bones in the arms, spine, hands, and feet (Shprintzen, 1997). Hand malformations caused by fusion usually involve the second, third, and fourth fingers, resulting in a claw-like appearance. The feet in Apert syndrome are usually normal, but in a few cases they will resemble hand malformations. Surgery is sometimes necessary on the hands and feet to improve function as well as cosmetic appearance.

Reports on cognitive function in Apert syndrome vary. Most resources report mental impairment as typical, ranging from learning disabilities to severe mental retardation. However, Gilbert (1996) cites a more positive prognosis, with 50% exhibiting mild learning disabilities while the other 50% demonstrate normal intelligence.

Behavioral Characteristics Profile . . . .

The behavioral characteristics associated with Apert syndrome are explained in this section.

Feeding and Breathing Problems

The facial features result in nasal abnormalities which can make it difficult or impossible for an infant to breathe while feeding. Nasogastric feeding is often necessary immediately after birth for several days to weeks. By 3-4 months, the problems gradually resolve with enlargement of the nasal passages through the normal growth process.

Developmental Delays

With Apert syndrome, it's important to follow development closely and to compare developmental milestones and neurological markers regularly. Any regression or decrease in the rate of physical or mental skills (as well as muscle tone in limbs) could indicate complicating factors such as hydrocephalus. If surgical intervention is required for syndrome features, hospitalizations may further impact the rate of normal development.

Learning Disability/Mental Retardation

Cognitive function can be impaired. Reports vary from normal intelligence to severe mental retardation on the intelligence continuum. Academic precursors should be monitored carefully to determine cognitive function and to begin appropriate educational stimulation as soon as necessary.

Cleft Palate and Dental Anomalies

A reported 30% of individuals have clefts of the soft palate and associated resonance problems. An open-bite malocclusion and crowded teeth further complicate development of articulation and vocal quality.

Conductive Hearing Loss

Craniofacial abnormalities typical in Apert syndrome also affect development of the middle ear. The conductive mechanisms for hearing are often bilaterally malformed. Space in the middle ear cavity is often reduced. Sound conduction is further impacted by fixation of the footplate of the stapes bone in the ossicular chain.

Speech-Language Delays

The development of speech and language is affected by many of the features. Cognitive function will influence language development most directly while structural deviations and hearing involvement will directly impact development of sound and vocal production abilities.

Speech-Language Issues . . . .

Speech-language development can be significantly impacted during early development by the features of Apert syndrome. Most of the difficulties experienced are secondary to primary features of the syndrome and should resolve satisfactorily with intervention, depending on the severity of the primary cause.

Articulation Delays

Errors in sound production are secondary to structural anomalies and cognitive ability. Most children with Apert syndrome have upper airway obstructions in the nasal passage that can interfere with oral/nasal airflow for consonant articulation. Cleft palate and malocclusions further compromise sound production. Depending on the severity of occlusion abnormalities, compensatory postures may be necessary for some consonant productions. The lower jaw can be large in Apert syndrome, and an open-bite posture is frequently evidenced.

Intervention Issues

- Articulation

- Voice

- Language

- Hearing

- Team Approach

Structural deviations in velar control for valving airflow and consonant production are also complicating factors. Cognitive function can impact the ability to learn sound production skills, but usually only if severe mental retardation is present.

Nasal Resonance Differences

Appropriate balance in nasal resonance is a problem in Apert syndrome. Hyponasality can occur from nasal obstructions and can be caused secondarily to cleft palate. The result is usually a mixed resonance problem.

Vocal Quality Differences

Vocal quality problems like hoarseness and breathiness can occur secondary to structural anomalies. Too much tension to overcome velopharyngeal valving difficulties can result in hoarseness, while poor control of airflow often results in breathiness.

Language Delays

Delays in language acquisition are generally secondary to the cognitive impairments. The possible brain anomalies of hydrocephalus and mental retardation will compromise the ability to acquire language structures and meaning. The delays will correlate to the severity of brain/cognitive involvement.

Conductive Hearing Loss

A conductive hearing loss usually has the greatest impact on articulation, not language. Hearing levels are usually functional and compensation is possible with hearing aids, if necessary. Hearing should be monitored to determine the degree of loss and impact it's likely to have on speech-language development over time, especially during the preschool language acquisition period.

Intervention for Apert syndrome will focus on deficits which occur secondarily in the disorder. Early intervention can dramatically improve a child's acquisition of basic language and motor skills when initiated as soon as possible following diagnosis.

Articulation

- Teach articulation of specific sounds using an oral-motor approach for correctly positioning the articulators.

- Consider using compensatory movements and postures to improve articulation.

- Make goals consistent with structural possibilities. The organic component may prevent accurate production of some phonemes.

- Consider orthodontic intervention to accompany articulation intervention.

Voice

- Emphasize breath support and easy onset of phonation to prevent excessive tension when the client is trying to speak.

- Monitor vocal quality aspects for hoarseness and/or breathiness and teach appropriate vocal production skills.

- Mixed resonance problems create unique challenges. Both hyponasality and hypernasality can be present at different structural levels—hyponasality due to nasal obstructions and hypernasality due to difficulties with velopharyngeal closure. Reinforce resonance balance with palatal exercises to strengthen velopharyngeal closure.

- Make goals consistent with organic capabilities and take into account structural limitations. Surgical intervention may be necessary if tissue obstructions are present in the nasal passage.

Language

- Stimulate receptive and expressive language as early as possible.

- Overcome developmental delays with early intervention and focused introduction of foundation language skills.

- Mediate language level by the level of cognitive functioning. The degree of mental retardation will impact goals and targeted levels.

Hearing

- Provide amplification to compensate for conductive hearing impairment, if necessary.

- Note that sound production and vocal quality may be compromised by hearing difficulties.

- Use visual stimulation to enhance and clarify auditory input.

Team Approach

- An audiologist should monitor hearing levels and make recommendations regarding possible hearing aids to compensate for conductive hearing loss.

- A neurologist should monitor developmental milestones to ascertain the possibility of hydrocephalus if a growth slowdown or regression is noted.

- A psychologist can provide counseling to assist a child in coping with cosmetic differences of the syndrome, if necessary. As a child grows older, his/her self-consciousness regarding appearance can lead to withdrawal and social problems.

- Surgical intervention may be required for abnormal fusion of the skull and hand/feet malformations to improve function and appearance.

- A special education teacher will be necessary if learning disabilities or mental retardation compromise normal academic progress.

Summary . . . .

Apert syndrome is marked by premature fusion of the skull, resulting in a mis-shapen head with a prominent forehead and a flattened back of the head. Facial features include large, widely-spaced eyes; a small nose with flattened bridge; and webbed hands and feet. Other features can include hydrocephalus, cleft palate, conductive hearing loss, and cognitive impairments. The syndrome is considered to be rare and affects both males and females. Life expectancy is normal, but can be compromised if severe organic or central nervous system involvement is present.

Surgical intervention may be necessary for several of the major features. Possibilities include a shunt for hydrocephalus, repairs for premature skull fusion to accommodate brain growth, repair for cleft palate and/or malocclusions, and modifications for function and appearance of hands and feet. Additional limitations might be imposed by mental disabilities.

Counseling may be necessary to address emotional aspects. The unusual facial features can lead to teasing and ridicule by peers, resulting in social isolation, withdrawal, or behavior problems. An added complication that occurs frequently is severe acne problems during adolescence. Frequent hospitalization for surgical intervention during the preschool years can also create psychological problems.

Many of the speech-language issues are secondary to primary features of Apert syndrome. Therefore, early intervention is critical and can significantly improve prognosis when initiated as soon as possible.

● ● ● ● ● ● ●

References . . . .

Batshaw, M. & Perret, Y. *Children with Disabilities—A Medical Primer, Third Edition.* Baltimore, MD: Paul H. Brookes Publishing Co., 1992.

Gilbert, P. *The A-Z Reference Book of Syndromes and Inherited Disorders, Second Edition.* New York, NY: Chapman & Hall, 1996.

Shprintzen, R. J. *Genetics, Syndromes, and Communication Disorders.* San Diego, CA: Singular Publishing Group, Inc., 1997.

●   ●   ●   ●   ●   ●   ●

Notes . . . .

Beckwith-Wiedemann Syndrome

Characteristics

- Macroglossia
- Dental problems
- Large stature
- Developmental delays
- Hypotonia

- umbilical abnormalities

- enlarged kidneys

- large growth pattern

- 7/100,000 live births

- hypoglycemia

- kidney tumors

- hypotonia

Syndrome Definition . . . .

Beckwith-Wiedemann syndrome is a relatively new syndrome. In 1963-1964, two physicians, Dr. Beckwith in America and Dr. Wiedemann in France, independently reported observing babies with certain, specific characteristics. Since then, numerous studies and reports have been generated on this particular syndrome.

Beckwith-Wiedemann syndrome is a genetic disorder whose characteristics are evident by ultrasound examination by the 20th week of pregnancy. Specific characteristics include a defective umbilicus and enlarged kidneys. Genetic inheritance is thought to be by autosomal dominant transmission, but most cases appear to be from a sporadic mutation. Incidence is approximately 7 in 100,000 live births, with males and females affected equally. Interestingly, a higher incidence (13 in every 700 births) is reported in the West Indies (Gilbert, 1996), but there is no explanation for this.

Umbilical abnormalities are evidenced at birth and can range in severity from small umbilical hernias to complete lack of closure in the anterior abdominal wall. Surgical intervention might be needed urgently, or may wait until the infant has matured enough to withstand operative trauma.

Babies with Beckwith-Wiedemann are abnormally large as evidenced by an above-average birth weight. Both height and weight tend to be in the upper 90th percentile on growth charts. The large size is also present in the growth rate of certain body organs, particularly the kidneys and adrenal glands. Occasionally, an excessive growth is seen in certain limbs. The accelerated growth rate tends to slow down after the early preschool years and subsides over time.

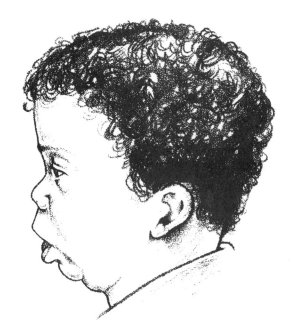

The overgrowth is thought to be responsible for hypoglycemia. The theory is that the insulin-producing cells in the pancreas are affected, resulting in problems with low blood sugar. Symptoms of hypoglycemia can include convulsions, breathing and feeding problems, lethargy, and cyanosis.

Children with Beckwith-Wiedemann are also prone to developing tumors of the kidney or adrenal glands. This problem is attributed to the overgrowth condition in the syndrome. Monitor children closely through childhood for any swelling or changes in the abdominal area that could signal the growth of a tumor. Surgical removal will determine the type of tumor (e.g., benign or malignant) and dictate necessity of postoperative treatments.

Facial characteristics of the syndrome include small noses, prominent eyebrows, and macrencephaly (large skull). Either earlobe may have an indentation or crease. This can aid in diagnosis of the syndrome. The most prominent facial anomaly is macroglossia, or an enlarged tongue, which generally protrudes from the mouth. The lower jaw may also be enlarged, resulting in a malocclusion.

A general hypotonia, or poor muscle tone, has been noted in babies. They are sometimes referred to as "floppy" babies because of the weak muscle tone and large size. Other problems associated with the syndrome include cleft lip and/ or palate, developmental delays due to cognitive impairment, and psychiatric/ behavioral problems.

The behavioral characteristics associated with Beckwith-Wiedemann syndrome are explained in the following section.

Macroglossia

The enlarged tongue in babies is usually apparent at birth. The tongue protrudes from the mouth and can create breathing problems if it falls back in the oral cavity, blocking air flow. As the child grows and facial structures enlarge, tongue size becomes less of a problem. Early intervention may help with facilitating feeding and breathing to prevent the tongue from falling in the oral cavity and blocking the passages for nutrition or air.

Dental Problems

The large tongue size can interfere with tooth eruption and alignment of the upper and lower jaw. An 'open bite' (when the child can't close his/her top and bottom teeth) is frequent in children suffering from the syndrome. An enlarged lower mandible is also common.

Large Stature

The largeness of children is most noticeable during the preschool years. Babies tend to put on weight quickly and grow at an above-average rate in both height and weight. The large size sometimes results in unrealistic expectations caused by a misinterpretation of developmental age.

Developmental Delays

Children with Beckwith-Wiedemann can be subject to general cognitive impairment, although generally mild in nature. Developmental milestones may be observed as delayed, and early intervention might be necessary to stimulate acquisition of language, motor, social, and academic skills.

Hypotonia

The poor muscle tone results in a floppy, lethargic appearance. Muscle coordination is further impaired by large structure size. Physical and occupational therapy are beneficial during the preschool years to promote increased muscle tone and coordination.

Speech-Language Issues

• Articulation

• Resonance

• Language

Speech-Language Issues . . . .

Speech-language problems occur because of a combination of low muscle tone, large tongue, and malocclusion due to an enlarged lower jaw. If a cleft component is present, features of the speech-language disorder like resonance, voice, and conductive hearing loss associated with cleft palate will increase.

Articulation

Production of speech is impaired by the large tongue and possible malocclusions due to open bite or large lower jaw. Compensatory postures may be necessary if clefts are also present. Oral muscle strength may be further impaired by weak muscle tone, resulting in imprecise articulatory postures.

Resonance

Balance of oral/nasal resonance can be compromised by several features. The large tongue structure may impair oral resonance. Poor muscle tone could result in hypernasality. Resonance and vocal quality can be impaired if a cleft lip and/or palate are present as part of the syndrome characteristics.

Language

Language development is only impaired if a cognitive deficit is present which impacts general language acquisition and development. Language aspects are usually mild and respond well to early intervention.

Intervention Issues . . . .

Speech-language issues in Beckwith-Wiedemann syndrome are relatively mild compared to many other syndromes evidenced in the preschool years. Most difficulties originate from the enlarged tongue and secondary complications of this structural anomaly; therefore, prognosis is good. Most deficits can be remediated to a functional, independent level.

Articulation

- Stimulate and directly target acquisition of sounds during preschool years. A motor approach might be the best approach because of the child's poor muscle control.

- Initiate oral-motor exercises to strengthen range of movement in the oral articulators, particularly coordinated tongue movement.

- Compensatory postures aren't necessary unless structural deviations are further impacted by aspects of cleft lip and/or palate.

Resonance

- Oral air pressure for sound production may be compromised by weak musculature and the large tongue. Velopharyngeal closure may be compromised by weak musculature due to hypotonia. Conduct exercises to strengthen velopharyngeal valving to improve appropriate oral/nasal airflow.

Language

- Stimulate language development in areas negatively impacted by any cognitive impairments. Address receptive and expressive language aspects at the same time.

- Address language deficits at the same time as academic readiness skills to prevent later school failure or difficulties.

Team Approach

- An orthodontist will need to treat dental anomalies and address issues in connection with malocclusions, such as an open bite.

- Surgical intervention will be necessary for significant umbilical abnormalities, such as umbilical hernias. Monitor the child carefully for any tumors in the abdominal wall and/or kidneys.

- Involve physical and occupational therapists early to help with problems associated with hypotonia.

- Teach parents the importance of specific sleeping postures that prevent respiratory blockage in infants, such as sleeping on one's side.

- Involve special education teachers if any cognitive impairments are present that have compromised academic achievement.

Summary . . . .

Beckwith-Wiedemann syndrome children are large at birth and may have large tongues, umbilical abnormalities, hypertonia, and creases in the earlobes. Growth is accelerated in physical structures and organs, which can lead to enlarged kidneys, liver, and spleen. Associated features can include possible cognitive impairments, heart anomalies, and hypoglycemia. Developmental tumors can occur in the abdominal wall and kidneys throughout childhood.

Early intervention and the child's responsiveness to therapy are good predictors of eventual functioning level. A normal life span is expected as long as there are no malignant tumors. Remediation should be very effective in

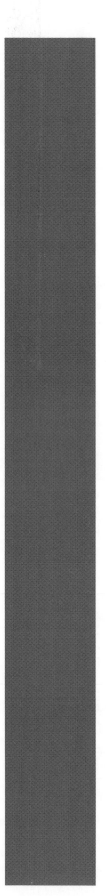

resolving most of the aspects of the syndrome. Academic deficits are generally mild and only compromised if cognitive impairment has occurred within the syndrome features. While surgical interventions may be necessary during the preschool years, significant complications do not usually occur. Prognosis and long-term options should be relatively normal, depending on the severity of the syndrome.

•   •   •   •   •   •   •

References

Gilbert, P. *The A-Z Reference Book of Syndromes and Inherited Disorders, Second Edition.* New York, NY: Chapman & Hall, 1996.

Shprintzen, R. J. *Genetics, Syndromes, and Communication Disorders.* San Diego, CA: Singular Publishing Group, Inc., 1997.

CHARGE Syndrome

Characteristics

- Hearing loss
- Resonance disorders
- Articulation impairments
- Language impairments
- Cognitive impairments
- Visual impairments

- **C**oloboma of the eye

- **H**eart defects

- **A**tresia of the choanae

- **R**etarded growth and development

- **G**enital abnormalities

- **E**ar anomalies and hearing loss/ deafness

Syndrome Definition · · · · · · · · · · ·

In regard to medical terminology, CHARGE syndrome is relatively new. In 1979, a physician noticed an associated group of symptoms that occurred at the same time as a defect in the nasal passage called choanal atresia. In 1986, it was suggested that the condition be called a syndrome rather than association of defects (Gilbert, 1996).

CHARGE is an acronym of the main deficits associated with the syndrome (see the acronym on the left). At least *two* of these primary features must be present for diagnosis.

- **Coloboma of the eye** is a failure of the retina or iris to fuse normally. This failure causes one or a number of parts/structures of the eye to be missing, such as a gap in the retina or other vital structure of the eye. The whole eye structure may be smaller, or the eyelids might be affected. The actual effect on vision will vary according to the type of deficit. It's estimated that 80% of children with CHARGE syndrome will have coloboma of the eye.

- **Heart defects** are variable in type and severity. However, any baby born with choanal atresia should be carefully examined for signs of heart deficits because the two conditions frequently occur together.

- **Atresia of the choanae** is a membranous or bony blockage (either unilateral or bilateral) of the nasal passage. If both sides are involved or if the blockage is severe, surgery is necessary to prevent potentially lethal respiratory problems. A defect of choanal atresia can be a life-threatening condition for an infant because babies breathe through their noses. The defect is sometimes not noticed until the child experiences his first upper-respiratory tract infection.

- **Retarded growth** occurs in 80% of babies with CHARGE syndrome. Weight and length parameters at birth are usually normal but have slowed considerably by six months of age.

- **Genital abnormalities** are usually characterized as hypoplasia, or small genital growth. Males are noted to have small penises.

- **Ear anomalies** are not always present but can occur with a variety of features. The earlobe may be triangular or it may be very small. Hearing loss can range from a mild loss to profound deafness. Both conductive and sensorineural losses occur. It is fairly common for children to exhibit a combined or mixed hearing loss.

CHARGE syndrome's etiology is unknown. It is considered a rare disorder. Due to the recency of the diagnosis, under 100 cases have been cited in incidence figures. Twice as many males are affected as females. It is not hereditary and recurrence risk in families is rare since it is considered to occur by sporadic mutation. Both autosomal dominant and recessive modes of inheritance have been described (Gilbert, 1996), and some cases have recently been linked to deletion of the long arm of chromosome 22 (Shprintzen, 1997).

Other features of CHARGE can include facial feature deficits such as facial asymmetry, small lower jaw, cleft lip and/or palate, facial paresis, and feeding disorders. The occurrence of cleft lip and/or palate increases other associated problems. For example, 50-90% of individuals with cleft palate are susceptible to severe persistent middle ear infections. More than 30% of children with cleft palate develop conductive hearing loss, and an additional 25% have sensorineural or a mixed type of hearing loss (Northern & Downs, 1991). Cognitive deficits have also been cited, ranging from learning disabilities to mental retardation.

A variety of other features (both educational and medical) can occur as primary or secondary symptoms of the syndrome. An actual case (female) diagnosed at age five evidenced the following physical symptoms in her medical profile of CHARGE syndrome: heart disease, multiple ear infections and bilateral conductive hearing loss, gastrointestinal problems, pneumonia, urinary tract infections, seizures, cleft lip and palate, sleep apnea, facial paralysis, facial asymmetry (nasal area), failure to thrive, asthma/allergies, and velopharyngeal inadequacy. Other characteristics will be noted in each section to illustrate the secondary impact of this complex syndrome profile.

Behavioral Characteristics Profile . . . .

The behavioral characteristics associated with CHARGE syndrome are explained in the following section.

Hearing Loss

Conductive and/or sensorineural (mixed) hearing loss (ranging from mild to severe) is common. The hearing impairment is further compounded by structural deviations that may also be present. For example, ossicular anomalies are possible in the middle ear. The abnormal structures associated with cleft palate can result in frequent otitis media, necessitating myringotomy to drain fluid from the middle ear. These complications, which cause significant conductive hearing problems, can be further compounded by a sensorineural loss. The hearing loss can have a secondary effect on language acquisition and pre-academic readiness skills.

Resonance Disorders

Several variables associated with CHARGE syndrome have a profound impact on achieving appropriate resonance in vocal production. One big factor is the occurrence of cleft palate, which results in hypernasality. Velopharyngeal incompetence also contributes to an excess of nasal resonance in the voice. The opposite can also be true. Choanal atresia (blockage in nasal passage) would result in hyponasality or an inability to accomplish nasal resonance.

Articulation Impairments

Articulation deficits are very common and can be rather complex due to the variety of factors which result in compromising sound production capability. For example, velopharyngeal inadequacy will result in articulation problems. The structural deficits associated with cleft lip and palate also cause significant impairment in articulation, including compensatory postures due to structural deficits. A third feature of CHARGE syndrome which results in articulation problems is facial paresis, or muscular weakness resulting in minimal positioning of the articulators.

Language Impairments

Difficulties in language acquisition are secondary to the primary features. Cognitive impairments will have an impact on receptive and expressive language development. Hearing loss will also negatively impact the onset of speech. A third, more subtle factor is the result of the intense medical interventions necessary during the developmental years. Frequent hospitalization and surgery will slow general development because the body must constantly engage in healing.

Cognitive Impairments

Global developmental delays are typical, secondary to cognitive impairment. Cognitive deficits can range from learning disabilities to levels of mental retardation. The impaired cognitive development will impact general acquisition of developmental milestones, including gross motor, fine motor, and adaptive behaviors.

Visual Impairments

Visual problems are possible in conjunction with the variety of facial anomalies. The structural deviations caused by the lack of fusion (coloboma) will vary in severity and impact, but the vast majority of those with the syndrome will evidence the visual deficits of the disorder. Visual acuity and structures should be checked during preschool years and appropriate modifications addressed in educational programming.

The female case example shared earlier had marked delays in development. For example, she did not sit alone until 12 months of age, she walked at two years, and she did not talk in short phrases until approximately five years. Despite the intellectual impairment, she was an active, energetic, and ambitious child with a delightful sense of humor and positive attitude!

Speech-Language Issues . . . .

Before beginning discussion of specific speech-language issues, here's a portion of an oral-peripheral examination in a diagnostic case report. This helps illustrate the scope of problems facing the clinician working with a child who has CHARGE.

Visual observation revealed a repaired unilateral cleft lip and palate. Teeth were misaligned with upper central incisors appearing intact. The left lateral incisor was present, however the right lateral incisor was absent. Tongue structure appeared normal in size, shape, muscle strength, and control. Soft palate was repaired.

Palate was pinkish in color with a high narrow contour. The uvula was deviated to the right side and appeared to demonstrate minimal elevation while producing /ah/. The nasal septum appeared to be asymmetrical and somewhat deviated, with the left nostril smaller in size as compared to the right nostril. Resonance quality was periodically noted as being denasal. Phonation demonstrated a dysphonic hoarse quality. The laryngeal valve appeared to be disrupted, compromising intelligibility of speech.

Restricted respiration resulted in a restricted voiced phonation time. During phonation of /ah/, the laryngeal valve continued to "shut on and off" with the majority of phonation consisting of the exhalation of remaining air with no accompanying voicing. Additional observations included the absence of tonsils, presence of a normal gag reflex, and no apparent restriction in the lingual frenum.

Articulation

Learning to correctly produce various vowels and consonants can be a challenge for children with CHARGE . As mentioned before, the articulation difficulties can be a secondary effect of several of the featured deficits. Typical error patterns include devoicing, final consonant

Speech-Language Issues

• Articulation

• Resonance

• Voice

• Hearing

• Language

omissions, substitution errors, and difficulty with plosives. The combination of hearing loss, cleft lip and palate, possible facial paresis, and nasal obstructions results in groups of errors which might be better approached through phonological intervention or by targeting groups by place, manner, or voicing in traditional articulation methods. Structural deviations might also necessitate compensatory postures to accomplish sound approximations.

Resonance

Accomplishing appropriate resonance may not be a realistic goal in CHARGE syndrome due to the multiple factors contributing to the problem. Most variables result in hypernasality issues from cleft palate, facial paresis, and velopharyngeal incompetency. However, if nasal passage obstructions have not been surgically addressed, hyponasality could be the primary concern. Again, the structural capabilities will dictate whether a balanced resonance can be achieved, but the primary goal should be to functionally enhance intelligibility. A significant hearing loss can also contribute to resonance problems.

Voice

Vocal quality can be compromised at the initial level of breath support for phonation due to paresis. Velopharyngeal incompetency and cleft palate can contribute to poor oral air pressure for sustained voicing. Common issues are a hoarse vocal quality and difficulty with sustained voicing. Hearing loss may add to the confusion of discriminating voiced vs. unvoiced consonants and final consonants.

Hearing

A mixed hearing loss of conductive components paired with sensorineural can significantly compromise hearing acuity in children with CHARGE syndrome. Ongoing

31

hearing infections from structural deviations common in cleft cases can lead to fluctuating hearing levels during preschool years of language and sound acquisition. Structural deviations, such as ossicular deformities, are also possible. The type and degree of hearing loss will greatly influence the impact it has on speech-language and academic learning.

Language

Language delay is common, but will be consistent with the cognitive impairment following preschool intervention. During early childhood years, it's important to stimulate language in very focused, intense intervention to overcome the developmental delays that occur routinely from the complications. Even children with minimal cognitive impairment will significantly lag behind developmental norms in the preschool years. The additional disadvantage of hearing loss will also impacts language acquisition.

Intervention Issues . . . .

Intervention for CHARGE syndrome will focus on deficits secondary to the primary features of the disorder. While the syndrome is complex, many of the aspects are medical and can be surgically corrected to a functional level. Therefore, intervention results can be very positive in their impact and significantly improve prognosis.

Articulation

• Evaluate and address production of specific sounds (e.g., stop-plosives, fricatives, and final consonants).

• Teach motor patterns for sounds, especially if structural variations or compensatory postures are necessary.

- Enhance discrimination of sound features through visual-tactile methods (e.g., mirror, blowing out candles, feeling vibrations) if hearing loss prevents normal sound field acuity for production discrimination.

Voice

- Teach sustained, controlled respiratory support for phonation to accomplish sustained voicing by using visual aids like balloons for blowing up, bubbles, etc.

- Practice and drill vowel prolongations to accomplish sustained voicing, then gradually expand to words, phrases, sentences, and conversation.

- Initiate exercises to strengthen velopharyngeal closure to address consonant production and resonance variables in speech production.

- Address resonance if structural deviations have been corrected. Teach discrimination of nasal resonance. Introduce exercises to strengthen oral vs. nasal air flow to accomplish better resonance balance.

Language

- Introduce and address receptive and expressive semantic vocabulary intensively during preschool years to build developmental language.

- Teach basic conceptual terms to build academic readiness skills.

- Note that language delays will be influenced by cognitive, hearing, and visual levels of performance.

Hearing

- Use hearing aids to compensate for conductive components and to enhance functional hearing.

- Introduce visual and tactile communication systems to compensate when hearing loss is significant or profound.

Team Approach

- Have an audiologist examine and monitor hearing levels, particularly for fluctuating conductive losses associated with otitis media common in cleft cases.

- Choanal atresia must be surgically corrected, especially if it's bilateral.

- Heart defects must be treated if present.

- Cleft lip and/or palate will require surgical repair.

- Vision must be checked in early childhood and monitored for changes. Significant deficits will require academic modifications.

- Special education teachers will be necessary to supplement academic learning at the appropriate cognitive level, ranging from learning disability to levels of mental retardation.

- Involve educational specialists with training in visual impairments for educational consultation and modifications. Also involve educational specialists with training in hearing impairments for consultation and modifications in the school setting.

- Counseling may be necessary to help the child cope with the multiple aspects of the disorder throughout the school years.

Summary . . . .

CHARGE syndrome is a disorder whose acronym represents its primary features:

Coloboma of the eye (failure of normal fusion of eye structures)
Heart defects
Atresia of choanae (blockage of nasal passages)
Retarded growth
Genital abnormalities
Ear anomalies and hearing loss

Additional deficits can include cleft lip and/or palate, velophargngeal inadequacy, facial paresis and asymmetry, gastrointestinal problems, and cognitive impairment.

Prognosis will depend on the severity of the cognitive and sensory deficits, but effective early intervention can have a tremendous impact on this disorder. The choanal atresia and heart problems present the most immediate and serious concerns. However, if dealt with adequately, the child should have a normal life expectancy.

Despite the significant and complex variety of symptoms in CHARGE syndrome, many of the problems can be surgically remediated during early childhood. Deficits in hearing, vision, and learning can affect future career options, but can be specifically addressed and compensated for in intervention. The little girl whose case example was used in this chapter responded very well to intervention efforts. By eight years of age, she was demonstrating receptive and expressive language skills of an age equivalency of six years (because of the cognitive impairment). She was doing well in school with supplemental services and was an outgoing, delightful student enjoyed by both teachers and peers.

●　　　●　　　●　　　●　　　●　　　●　　　●

References

Batshaw, M. & Perret, Y. *Children with Disabilities—A Medical Primer, Third Edition.* Baltimore, MD: Paul H. Brookes Publishing Co., 1992.

Gilbert, P. *The A-Z Reference Book of Syndromes and Inherited Disorders, Second Edition.* New York, NY: Chapman & Hall, 1996.

Northern, J. & Downs, M. *Hearing in Children, Fourth Edition.* Baltimore, MD: Williams & Wilkins, 1991.

Shprintzen, R. J. *Genetics, Syndromes, and Communication Disorders.* San Diego, CA: Singular Publishing Group, Inc., 1997.

Cri-du-Chat Syndrome

Characteristics

- Hypotonicity
- Mental retardation
- Low birth weight/Significant postnatal growth deficiency
- Self-injurious behavior

- "cry of the cat"

- 1/20,000 to 1/50,000 live births

- microcephaly

- mental retardation

- severe speech-language delays

- congenital heart defects

Syndrome Definition . . . .

Cri-du-Chat syndrome is caused by a partial chromosomal deletion on a segment of the short arm of the fifth chromosome (5p-). It was documented in the 1960s by Professor Lejeune and is also referred to as Lejeune syndrome. The most definitive characteristic of the syndrome is a high-pitched cry in infancy that sounds like the meowing of a cat. Thus the name of the syndrome literally means "cry of the cat" in French.

Incidence numbers vary from 1/20,000 to 1/50,000 live births (Pore & Reed, 1999; Batshaw, 1997; Gerber, 1998). The gender occurrence seems to be about equal, with a slightly higher incidence in girls than in boys. The syndrome can be identified at 9-12 weeks gestation through chorionic villus sampling or at 16 weeks through amniocentesis.

A high percentage of children are reported to have microcephaly (up to 98% according to Gilbert, 1996). It's reported that about 1% of all children with severe mental retardation have this syndrome (Gerber, 1998). Severe mental retardation (with intelligence quotients below 30 or 35) is reported for the majority of this population (Shprintzen, 1997; Gerber, 1998).

Children with Cri-du-Chat syndrome exhibit severely deficient speech-language skills, and many develop no speech at all. If speech does develop, onset is extremely delayed and the resulting articulation impairment is severe. The language involvements are equivalent to the cognitive-functioning level. Hearing is not reported to be a significant concern unless a conductive loss is noted secondary to chronic otitis media.

Many specific physical anomalies are associated with the syndrome. A broad face with widely-spaced, downward slanting eyes is a common appearance. Microcephaly, facial asymmetry, dental malocclusions, a prominent nasal root, and micrognathia are reported. Low-set, posteriorly-rotated ears are seen, and ear tags may also be present. Eye characteristics include strabismus, myopia, and a divergent squint.

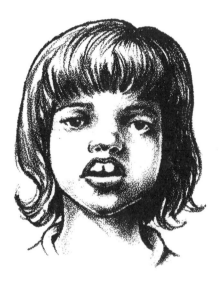

Congenital heart defects are noted in one-third of these children, particularly patent ductus arteriosus. Absence of the kidney and spleen, inguinal hernia, malrotation of the large bowel, club or flat feet, and hip dislocations may occur. Severe hypotonicity affects development of ambulation, feeding, and respiration abilities. Life span is low because of the many cardiac and respiratory difficulties, but many children live to be adults.

Behavioral Characteristics Profile . . . .

The behavioral characteristics associated with Cri-du-Chat syndrome are explained in the following section.

Hypotonicity

Severe hypotonia is reported in these children. This lack of muscle tone affects many of the systems in the developing child, including the respiratory system, the feeding system, and physical development. Severe breathing difficulties result from the hypotonicity and are further complicated by the small size of the respiratory passages. Failure to thrive due to the severity of feeding difficulties can occur. You may have to introduce tube feeding in order to maintain adequate nutrition. Slow physical development, including head control and ambulation, is common.

Speech-Language Issues

- High-Pitched Cry

- Cleft Lip and/or Palate

- Severe Receptive and
  Expressive Language
  Impairments

- Hearing

Mental Retardation

Severe mental retardation is noted, with reported intelligence quotients not reaching above 30 to 35. Microcephaly can cause this lack of cognitive development. As development progresses, the cognitive deficits become more apparent. One percent of children with severe mental retardation are estimated to be affected by Cri-du-Chat syndrome. The severity of the mental retardation indicates that members of this population will not lead independent lives and will need extensive support.

Low Birth Weight/ Significant Postnatal Growth Deficiency

Children with the syndrome are small at birth and can exhibit failure to thrive due to feeding difficulties. A significant postnatal growth deficiency is also present, resulting in short stature.

Self-Injurious Behavior

Self-injurious behavior and repetitive movements have been reported. In addition to these physical behaviors, hypersensitivity to sensory stimulation has also been noted.

Speech-Language Issues . . . .

Speech-language issues in Cri-du-Chat are associated with the small size of various structures, hypotonicity, and severe mental retardation. The predominant existence of microcephaly and mental retardation in the population affects the development of both speech and language skills.

High-Pitched Cry

The high-pitched cry (compared to that of a meowing cat) heard in infancy is a noted characteristic of the syndrome. Most studies say the cry is caused by hypoplasia and small size of the laryngeal structure. It's reported that as the larynx grows, the high-pitched cry is lost.

Cleft Lip and/or Palate

Complete lack of speech development is not uncommon. If speech does develop, hypernasality and compensatory articulation errors may be noted if a cleft lip or cleft palate are present. The oral cavity may be extremely narrow, which also affects articulation. A high-pitched voice may continue, as in the infant cry. Severe delay in onset of speech and vast articulatory impairment may also occur, resulting from neurological causes. Echolalic speech has also been reported. Consider augmentative and alternative means of communication for those who do not develop functional speech.

Severe Receptive and Expressive Language Impairments

If language skills do develop, they are apt to be rudimentary or primitive. Augmentative and alternative means of communication should be investigated to allow children to communicate their wants and needs. The language development that does occur will be limited by the cognitive deficiencies.

Hearing

Hearing abilities are reported as an area of less concern. A conductive hearing loss, secondary to chronic otitis media, is the most often reported complication for hearing.

Intervention Issues

- Feeding and Respiration

- Augmentative and Alternative Communication

- Team Approach

Intervention Issues . . . .

Intervention for Cri-du-Chat syndrome centers around the severity of structural and cognitive deficiencies.

Feeding and Respiration

- Feeding intervention is recommended due to the small size of the infant and because of respiration and hypotonia. Consultation with the family and an occupational therapist (if necessary) will allow you to develop a feeding protocol. Tube feeding may also be necessary for adequate nutritional intake.

Augmentative and Alternative Communication

- Introduce augmentative and alternative communication methods early in the child's life. Encourage early gestures and signs with family/caregiver support.

- For those children who develop some true symbolic ability, design a communication board, book, or electronic communication device.

Team Approach

- Early intervention is essential. Language stimulation, centering around caregiver-child interactions, should begin as soon as the child is medically stable. Use additional stimulation in the areas of verbal, auditory, and visual senses for cognitive growth.

- Consult with a surgeon about early repair of structural abnormalities such as cleft lip or palate, or heart.

- Early intervention and early childhood special education will promote cognitive and social growth.

- Medical interventionists should monitor low birth weight and respiratory difficulties and recommend needed surgeries for structural repair.

- Consult with an audiologist in cases of chronic otitis media or suspected hearing loss.

- Consult with an occupation therapist about feeding difficulties and hypotonia.

- A physical therapist is valuable because body development is atypical and activities for gross and fine motor skills may be needed.

- Make the child's family the nucleus of the team because they are the primary caregivers and interactional partners of the child.

Summary • • • • • • • • • • • • • • • • • • •

Cri-du-Chat syndrome is a genetic disorder caused by a partial deletion of the short arm of chromosome 5. Severe hypotonia, severe mental retardation with microcephaly, and significant developmental impairments are found. Children affected by this syndrome will need extensive support and are not expected to lead independent lives.

There are many physical complications. Structural differences causing early respiration and feeding difficulties are the most life-threatening. Small birth weight, failure to thrive, and congenital heart defects put children at further risk.

Speech may not develop in these children, and if it develops at all, it may be severely impaired. Causes for the speech difficulties can be neurological or structural (e.g., clefts, narrow oral cavity formation). Language is severely impaired in both the receptive and expressive areas. The language that does develop will be affected by the cognitive deficiencies. Use augmentative and alternative means of communication on a case-by-case basis.

Early intervention with a team approach is highly recommended. Medical, educational, and therapeutic interventions may all be necessary for a child to progress to his or her maximum level of abilities.

References

Batshaw, M. L. *Children with Disabilities, Fourth Edition.* Baltimore, MD: Paul H. Brookes Publishing Co., 1997.

Gerber, S. E. *Etiology and Prevention of Communicative Disorders, Second Edition.* San Diego, CA: Singular Publishing Group, Inc., 1998.

Gilbert, P. *The A-Z Reference Book of Syndromes and Inherited Disorders, Second Edition.* New York, NY: Chapman & Hall, 1996.

Pore, S. G. & Reed, K. L. *Quick Reference to Speech-Language Pathology.* Gaithersburg, MD: Aspen Publishers, Inc., 1999.

Shprintzen, R. J. *Genetics, Syndromes, and Communication Disorders.* San Diego, CA: Singular Publishing Group, Inc., 1997.

Notes . . . .

Crouzon Syndrome

Characteristics

- Psychosocial problems
- Normal cognition

- premature fusion of skull and facial bones

- severe midface deformities

- protruding eyeballs

- tooth overcrowding

Syndrome Definition . . . .

Crouzon syndrome is a congenital defect that is also known as craniofacial dysostosis (McWilliams et al., 1990). The skull and facial skeletons are primarily affected by premature fusion (craniosynostosis), specifically, the coronal and saggital sutures of the skull plates. This skull fusion can restrict brain growth, cause severe midface deformities, and affect the relationship of the teeth. Increased intracranial pressure and abnormal head shape are also exhibited. Severity of the deformity varies from person to person, and depends on when the fusion process begins and how quickly it progresses.

The syndrome is caused by a defect in the fibrobast growth factor receptor-2, found on the long arm of chromosome 10, and is an autosomal dominant genetic condition. Genetic counseling is recommended for those considering reproducing. The syndrome was first identified by Dr. Crouzon.

The top of the head and the forehead are flattened. A short cranial base is common with the anterior base shortened and the angulation of the skull base acute (kyphosis). This can rotate the skull clockwise, which pushes the posterior skull base forward and the forehead back (Shprintzen, 1997). Agenesis of the corpus collosum has also been noted.

Visual disturbances occur in Crouzon syndrome. Shallow orbits and proptosis (protruding eyeballs) are seen in addition to strabismus and nystagmus. Hypertelorism (an increased separation of the entire orbit including its contents) is common (Shprintzen, 1997). Optic nerve defects occur in approximately 80% of cases, and other eye anomalies may be present. Exorbitism (eyes that bulge from their orbits) is also exhibited.

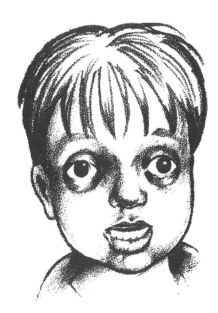

The midface deformities include severe maxillary hypoplasia, which results in a protruding jaw and overcrowding of the maxillary teeth. The midface area may have a sunken look. A class III malocclusion can occur as a result of lower teeth occluding the upper teeth. A narrow, high-arched palate; occasional cleft of the palate; and a short upper lip are also noted. A short, beaked nose is exhibited and severely reduced nasal airways coincide. The oropharynx may be shallow, resulting in mouth-breathing behaviors. A long, thin velum may block the nasaopharyngeal area.

Behavioral Characteristics Profile . . . .

The behavioral characteristics associated with Crouzon syndrome are explained in the following section.

Psychosocial Problems

Psychosocial problems are directly related to the skull and facial appearances. Social isolation, restricted vocational and lifemate choices, and the anxiety of producing children all play a part in social development.

Normal Cognition

If the craniosynostosis and intracranial pressure are managed early in the client's life, then typical cognitive growth is expected. Any cognitive deficiencies will be determined by the amount of brain dysfunction. Occasional seizure disorders are also noted.

Speech-Language Issues . . . .

Many children with Crouzon develop speech and language within normal limits. Communication difficulties are affected by the degree of palatal involvement, cognitive function, severity of oral cavity anomalies, and type and degree of hearing loss.

Hearing Loss

One-third to one-half of those with Crouzon syndrome experience hearing loss. These are generally nonprogressive, conductive hearing losses, and can result from a variety of causes. Absence of ear canals, deformities of the middle ear, absence or unusual positioning of tympanic membranes, or hypoplasticity of the tympanic membranes can all occur, as well as ossicular chain fixation. Eustachian tube dysfunction has also been noted. Sensorineural losses can also be exhibited, but with less frequency. Meniere's disease has also been reported.

Articulation Disorders

Articulation impairment is common because of the midface hypoplasia. The Class III malocclusion (with mandibular protrusion) will affect articulation, depending on the severity of the deformity. Mild mandibular protrusion may cause no difficulty in producing speech, while more evident deformity will affect the lingua-alveolars, sibilants, fricatives, and affricates. Crossbite and/or open bite can further complicate mandibular protrusion and the production of phonemes. This oral cavity misalignment is a prominent factor in articulation production.

Resonance Disorders

The severity of the craniofacial and skull deformities will affect resonance. Hyponasal resonance may be heard due to the shallow oropharynx (a small nasal capsule) and the presence of a thick, elongated palate. Hypernasal speech will accompany any palatal cleft and you may also hear nasal emission.

Language Development

Language development parallels cognitive function. If early intervention and early surgeries permit typical brain growth and relieve intracranial pressure, then language should develop within normal limits. Cognitive impairments are not typical. The type and degree of hearing loss may also affect language development.

Intervention Issues

Intervention Issues . . . .

Determine intervention for Crouzon syndrome by looking at the severity of the skull and midface deformities; the beginning and progression of the craniosynostosis; and its affect on breathing, feeding, hearing, vision, and brain development. A complete evaluation of the child and the intervention of a craniofacial team is highly recommended.

Hearing

- Early surgical reconstruction of the outer or middle ear may be necessary.

- Treat the conductive loss from an otological approach with attention to chronic otitis media.

- Use amplification if necessary.

Speech

- Early identification and early intervention is essential.

- Early surgery may enhance articulation development and voice production.

- Provide traditional articulation therapy for sibilants, fricatives, and affricates.

- Reduce nasal emissions. Make the child aware of the difference between oral cavity production and nasal cavity production.

Language

- Provide the child with language stimulation for maximum cognitive development.

Team Approach

- Audiologists can help the high percentage of those with hearing loss.

- Consider a craniofacial team composed of an ear, nose, and throat doctor; neurosurgeon; plastic surgeon; and orthodontist.

- Include the child's family as team members.

- Psychologists, teachers, or social workers can also serve on the team to deal with psychosocial disorders associated with the facial deformities.

- Include ophthalmologic services to treat visual difficulties.

Summary ·

Crouzon syndrome is a congenital defect also known as craniofacial dysostosis. It is primarily concerned with craniosynostosis, a premature fusion of the sutures of the skull that results in skull deformities and severe midface anomalies. Breathing, feeding, vision, hearing, and brain development disorders are all associated with the syndrome.

A team approach is highly recommended: speech-language pathologists, audiologists, medical personnel, and psychologists may all be called upon for services. Multiple surgeries are not uncommon.

References

Batshaw, M. L. *Children with Disabilities, Fourth Edition.* Baltimore, MD: Paul H. Brookes Publishing Co., 1997.

"Crouzon Syndrome Information." <http://www.crouzon.org/crouzon.html/> July 14, 1999.

Gerber, S. E. *Etiology and Prevention of Communicative Disorders, Second Edition.* San Diego, CA: Singular Publishing Group, Inc., 1998.

Gilbert, P. *The A-Z Reference Book of Syndromes and Inherited Disorders, Second Edition.* New York, NY: Chapman & Hall, 1996.

McWilliams, B. J., Moris, H. L., & Shelton, R. L. *Cleft Palate Speech, Second Edition.* Philadelphia, PA: B. C. Decker, Inc., 1990.

Pore, S. G. & Reed, K. L. *Quick Reference to Speech-Language Pathology.* Gaithersburg, MD: Aspen Publishers, Inc., 1999.

Shprintzen, R. J. *Genetics, Syndromes, and Communication Disorders.* San Diego, CA: Singular Publishing Group, Inc., 1997.

Shprintzen, R. J. & Bardach, J. *Cleft Palate Speech Management: A Multidisciplinary Approach.* St. Louis, MO: Mosby, 1995.

Goldenhar Syndrome

Characteristics

- Hearing impairments
- Vision impairments
- Normal intelligence
- Emotional disorders

- anomalies in head, face, and neck areas

- 1/5,600 to 1/45,000 live births

- slightly higher rate in boys than in girls

- varying inheritance patterns

- "wide mouth"

Syndrome Definition . . . .

Goldenhar syndrome is a disorder identified by a wide spectrum of symptoms and a great variety of mild-to-profound physical features. The cause is unknown, and while a sporadic inheritance pattern is reported, there are several known familial cases, some of which have an apparent autosomal dominant or recessive transmission. A multifactorial inheritance of environment and genetics working together has been suggested.

There is a discrepancy in the incidence numbers reported, with a range from 1/5,600 to 1/45,000 live births (Jung, 1989; Pore & Reed, 1999). The syndrome occurs at a slightly higher rate in boys than in girls.

Goldenhar was first recognized as a specific pattern of malformation in 1952, but the full spectrum of anomalies was not fully recognized until the 1960s (Shprintzen, 1997). Although great variability is noted in the disorder, anomalies tend to affect certain sections of the head, face, and spinal column. The cheekbones, jaws, mouth, ears, eyes, and cervical bones of the spinal column are most likely to be affected.

Often the identified anomalies are asymmetrical and unilateral. If they are bilateral, the right side is typically more affected than the left in 10-33% of the cases (NORD, 1999). The syndrome is apparent at birth, and prenatal ultrasound has been successful in identifying severe ear abnormalities and skeletal abnormalities.

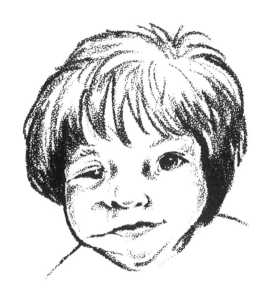

Outer ear anomalies include atresia (absent ear canals), anotia (absence of the outer ear), microtia (malformation of the outer ear), accessory ear tags, and preauricular pits (abnormal growths of skin and cartilage in front of or on the ears). The middle ear can be tiny or misshapen. The Eustachian tube may also be malformed.

Facial malformations can include hypoplasia of the maxilla or mandible, high-arched palate, crowded teeth, malocclusion, facial palsy, cleft palate or cleft lip and palate, and hemifacial microsomia (the face is smaller on one side than the other). The hemifacial microsomia is due to the underdevelopment of the mandibular ramus and condyle. The facial nerve can run an unusual course, thus paresis of the soft palate; and pharyngeal, palatal, and tongue asymmetry are common. Closed or absent nares have also been reported.

Unilateral macrostomia, or an abnormally "wide mouth," is reported in many cases. Jung (1989) refers to the lateral cleftlike extensions from the corner of the mouth that result in this apparent macrostomia. Commissural cleft is also used in this description.

The entire mandible tends to be underdeveloped (mandibular hypoplasia), although one side is worse than the other (Gerber, 1998). The more typically-developing side grows more rapidly than the other side. This results in a concavity in the abnormal side that gets gradually worse and intensifies the appearance of the facial asymmetry.

Eye abnormalities occur in about one-third of cases and include strabismus, eyelid clefts (coloboma), microphthalmia (smallness of the eye), anophthalmia (congenital absence of the eye), or cysts on the eyeball (ocular choristomas or dermoid cysts).

Other abnormalities include gastrointestinal disorders; renal (kidney) disorders; cardiac, neurological, and pulmonary involvement; and skeletal anomalies in the forearm and thumbs. Scoliosis may also be present. Life span is expected to be within normal limits if breathing obstructions and heart defects are corrected early in life.

Goldenhar Syndrome is also known as:

- Hemifacial Microsomia (HFM)
- Facialauriculovertebral Malformation Sequence (FAV)
- Oculo-Auriculo-Vertebral Dysplasia (OAV)
- First and Second Brachial Arch Syndrome
- Goldenhar-Gorlin Syndrome

Behavioral Characteristics Profile · · · · · · · · · · ·

The behavioral characteristics associated with Goldenhar syndrome are explained in the following section.

Hearing Impairments

Conductive hearing loss (usually unilateral) is most often seen in Goldenhar syndrome. This loss is congenital, as the malformations of the outer and middle ear can affect the conduction of sound. An occasional sensorineural loss is reported.

Vision Impairments

The effect of the craniofacial anomalies, particularly to the eye area, is significant in causing visual impairments. The possible smallness of the eye, cysts on the actual eyeball, and eyelid clefts are included in these anomalies. Strabismus has also been reported in the population.

Normal Intelligence

Most children with Goldenhar have normal intelligence. Those with cognitive challenges constitute only 5-15% of the population and are in the mild or educable range.

Emotional Disorders

Emotional disorders can occur for those with severely deformed faces. Multiple surgeries may be needed to repair and restructure various facial anomalies.

Speech-Language Issues

- Feeding Difficulties/ Dysphagia

- Hearing

- Resonance

- Articulation

- Oral Language

Speech-Language Issues . . . .

Speech-language issues within Goldenhar syndrome are primarily a result of the various anomalies. Early intervention upon diagnosis is critical, particularly in the areas associated with speech-language development.

Feeding Difficulties/Dysphagia

Dysphagia and failure to thrive are concerns because of upper-airway obstructions caused by mandibular and pharyngeal anomalies. The small, receding chin can specifically interfere with infant feeding. A cleft lip or a cleft lip and palate can also conflict with feeding. Tube feeding is not uncommon for infants for their nutritional needs. The oral-motor area may also be sensitive for these children, particularly after surgeries. For some children, feeding will be an anxious experience.

Hearing

A unilateral, conductive hearing loss is the most commonly reported hearing impairment. This loss is a result of the malformations seen in the outer ear and in the middle ear. An occasional bilateral conductive loss may

* Feeding/Dysphagia/
  Oral Sensitivity

* Hearing

* Voice

* Articulation

* Language

* Team Approach

occur which indicates an immediate need for amplification. Sporadic sensorineural loss has also been reported. Early identification of any existing hearing loss is critical to circumvent further speech-language developmental delays.

Resonance

The most common voice disorder is hypernasality which is secondary to pharyngeal asymmetry/clefting. Resonance production may also be affected by conductive or sensorineural hearing loss. Surgeries or prosthedontic treatment can modify vocal resonance. Hoarseness may also be present which might be due to unilateral vocal fold paralysis.

Articulation

Articulation deficits relate primarily to hearing loss and structural anomalies like cleft lip and palate. Asymmetrical tongue movement, malocclusion, and possible compensatory articulation movements associated with clefting have been observed. Conductive or sensorineural hearing loss will affect articulation production, especially if the loss is bilateral.

Oral Language

Oral language has been noted as an area of concern. Syntax, semantics, and pragmatics are all reported as deficits. Early intervention programs can target development of these skills.

Intervention in Goldenhar syndrome will rely heavily on a multidisciplinary, team approach. Surgeries for craniofacial malformations, speech-language and audiological services, and family/caregiver involvement are all crucial to the child's development. It's important to improve function and facial symmetry, and manage the structural malformations (Jung, 1989).

Feeding/Dysphagia/Oral Sensitivity

- Assess feeding and swallowing skills in infancy to insure that the child is receiving adequate nutrition. Conditions that affect feeding include cleft lip, cleft palate, and mandibular and pharyngeal malformations.

- Assess oral-area sensitivity and oral-motor adequacy for feeding.

- Develop a feeding program that includes parent/caregiver training.

- Facilitate reduction of oral hypersensitivity with play, exploration, and fun oral-sensory activities.

Hearing

- Hearing loss should be diagnosed early in the child's life. Ear anomalies may be seen at birth, and newborn screenings may identify the need for intervention. Early identification assists prevention of later speech-language disorders.

- Surgery may be a consideration to repair the outer ear or middle ear anomalies, if necessary. Also monitor Eustachian tube form and function.

- Provide or monitor amplification if a bilateral conductive loss is identified.

Voice

- Surgical repair may be needed for the maxillary areas and pharyngeal areas to improve oral and nasal resonance.

- Indicate easy onset and soft approach of vocalizing. Refer for medical treatment/evaluation in the event of hoarseness.

Articulation

- Surgical repair for cleft lip and/or palate to enhance articulatory production may be needed.

- Surgical repair for the jaw to increase the size of the underdeveloped mandible and to ease the movement of the mandible against the temporal bone may be needed. Use orthodontic treatment to redirect future growth.

- Initiate traditional articulation therapy and address developmentally appropriate sounds that follow specific assessments in this area.

Language

- Provide early intervention and emphasize oral-language development with a team approach.

- Encourage family and caregiver training to increase oral language production in areas like parallel talk, self-talk, expansions, and modeling.

- Use targeted objectives in older children that include areas of oral language production like semantics, syntax, and pragmatics.

- Periodically assess oral-language development.

Team Approach

- An audiologist should conduct testing of newborns and give periodic evaluations to monitor identified hearing loss or hearing fluctuations as the child develops.

- A craniofacial team needs to be medically involved. An ear, nose, and throat specialist can manage the structural malformations.

- A psychologist may need to be consulted for the child who develops emotional difficulties because of the severity of the malformations.

- As a speech-language pathologist, provide primary treatment for speech, language, hearing, and oral-motor issues.

- As the child faces surgical repair for optimum prognosis, make sure he or she interacts with all members of the craniofacial and educational teams, including the family or caregiver.

- A deaf educator may be added to the treatment team if hearing loss is significant.

- An occupational therapist may play a part in treatment if the child has significant oral sensitivity and feeding issues.

- An orthodontist may need to provide treatment for any malocclusions.

Summary · · · · · · · · · · · · · · · · · · ·

Goldenhar syndrome is a disorder identified by a wide variety of symptoms and a great diversity of physical features ranging in severity from mild to profound. A sporadic inheritance pattern is reported, but an actual cause is unknown. A multifactorial inheritance with environment and genetics combined has also been suggested. Incidence numbers range from 1/5,600 to 1/45,000 live births, with a slightly higher rate in boys than in girls.

Although great variability is noted in the disorder, anomalies tend to affect certain sections of the head and face area and the spinal column bones. The cheekbones, jaw, mouth, ears, and eyes, as well as the cervical bones of the spinal column are most commonly affected. These anomalies are often asymmetrical and unilateral, but if they are bilateral, the right side is typically more affected than the left. Goldenhar is apparent at birth.

Conductive, unilateral hearing loss is most often seen in Goldenhar syndrome. An occasional sensorineural loss is reported. The effect of the craniofacial anomalies (particularly to the eyes) is significant in causing visual impairments.

Most people with Goldenhar have normal intelligence. Those with cognitive challenges constitute only 5-15% of the population and they are in the mild or educable range. Emotional disorders may be more frequent in those with severely deformed faces.

Speech-language issues in Goldenhar are primarily a result of the various anomalies associated with the syndrome. Dysphagia and failure to thrive are concerns due to upper airway obstructions caused by mandibular and pharyngeal anomalies. Cleft lip, or cleft lip and palate, can disturb feeding movement and can affect voice and articulation. As far as voice disorders, hypernasality secondary to pharyngeal asymmetry or clefting is most common. Oral language is a particular area of concern.

Intervention will rely heavily on a multidisciplinary team approach. Surgeries for craniofacial malformations, speech-language and audiological services, and family involvement are all crucial to the child's development. Early intervention with an emphasis on oral language development is recommended, with emphasis on a team approach.

●   ●   ●   ●   ●   ●   ●

References

Batshaw, M. L. *Children with Disabilities, Fourth Edition.* Baltimore, MD: Paul H. Brookes Publishing Co., 1997.

Gerber, S. E. *Etiology and Prevention of Communicative Disorders, Second Edition.* San Diego, CA: Singular Publishing Group, Inc., 1998.

Gilbert, P. *The A-Z Reference Book of Syndromes and Inherited Disorders, Second Edition.* New York, NY: Chapman & Hall, 1996.

Jung, J. H. *Genetic Syndromes in Communication Disorders.* Austin, TX: Pro-Ed., 1989.

National Organization for Rare Disorders, Inc. (NORD). *Disease Information: Goldenhar Syndrome.* (Oculo Auriculo Vertebral Spectrum). July 12, 1999.

Pore, S. G. & Reed, K. L. *Quick Reference to Speech-Language Pathology.* Gaithersburg, MD: Aspen Publishers, Inc., 1999.

Shprintzen, R. J. *Genetics, Syndromes, and Communication Disorders.* San Diego, CA: Singular Publishing Group, Inc., 1997.

Klinefelter Syndrome

Characteristics

- Learning disabilities
- Mental retardation
- Poor coordination
- Delayed social development
- Behavior disorders

- occurs only in males

- 1/500 to 1/1000 men

- usually not detected until male is school-aged

- tallness and long limbs

- underdeveloped genitalia

- poor coordination

Syndrome Definition . . . .

Klinefelter syndrome is a common chromosomal variation found in males that causes a hormone imbalance and sterility. It is found in 1/500 to 1/1000 men. Though infertility is present, sexual function can be normal.

Klinefelter is diagnosed through a karotype, which is a chromosomal analysis done on a blood sample. The variation is an extra X sex chromosome in affected males. There are also less common variations of two, three, and four extra X chromosomes. The severity of associated features increases as the number of X chromosomes increases.

The syndrome was first described in 1942 by Dr. Harry Klinefelter and his colleagues who reported on men with similar physical patterns. The exact chromosomal makeup of the population was not determined until 1956. Older mothers have a slightly higher risk of bearing sons with Klinefelter syndrome but there are no other known risk factors. The syndrome is not usually identified in infants and it may not truly be diagnosed until a child enters school and learning difficulties are encountered. It may also be detected at puberty when secondary sex characteristics fail to emerge.

Affected males tend to be tall and slim with long limbs, underdeveloped male genitalia, and possible breast development. Characteristics of the syndrome (other than sterility) have been successfully treated with testosterone therapy in teens, adolescents, and adults. A normal life span is expected.

Behavioral Characteristics Profile . . . .

The primary behavioral characteristics associated with Klinefelter syndrome are explained in the following section.

Learning Disabilities

Clients with Klinefelter are at risk for learning problems. Many boys appear to exhibit attention deficit disorder. Dyslexia can also be a problem, particularly after puberty. Spatial skills have been noted to be strong particularly in music and art.

Mental Retardation

Males affected by Klinefelter syndrome may test in the range of mental retardation. Because they do not progress cognitively with their peers, a progressive mental retardation may be exhibited. Low to average intelligence has been reported, with verbal intelligence quotients being lower than performance intelligence quotients (Gerber, 1998).

Poor Coordination

Males with Klinefelter syndrome are tall (average height 6'1/2") with long limbs, poor coordination, and a general lack of athleticism. Hand tremors and intentional tremor are reported in 20-50% of the population (Batshaw, 1997).

Delayed Social Development

Characteristics can affect the social development of affected males, particularly self-esteem. They may be less confident in their maleness than other boys and may appear more immature. Shyness, a lack of initiative, and extreme sensitivity have all been reported. The nature of the shyness may make the child test less cognitively adept than he is.

Behavior Disorders

Clients suffering from Klinefelter syndrome may experience frustration. Outbursts are noted, as are lower levels of activity and endurance, and restless sleep patterns. Mental illness and an increased risk for diabetes have been reported in the adult population. (Batshaw, 1997).

Speech-Language Issues . . . .

Studies indicate that in Klinefelter syndrome, speech-language difficulties affect social behavior and learning.

Delayed Speech-Language Skills

Speech development may be at risk for boys with Klinefelter syndrome. Gerber (1998) reported that 75% of affected males have delays of language and phonological structures. Both receptive and expressive language skills are at risk (Pore & Reed, 1999). Articulation disorders may also be exhibited.

Language Processing Disorders

Language processing disorders and auditory memory problems are noted in the syndrome. The language processing disorder may be interpreted as a lack of language comprehension in various contexts.

Voice and Hearing

Voice use and production are within normal limits, although the expected lower voice pitch following puberty may be absent. Cleft palate is occasionally found. Hearing is generally within normal limits, with 20% of the population reported to have progressive hearing impairments (Gerber, 1998).

Intervention Issues . . . .

Intervention in Klinefelter syndrome will rely on hormone therapy and early intervention, especially curriculum-based intervention.

Hormone Therapy

• Currently, the most effective therapy for Klinefelter syndrome is testosterone therapy. Testosterone has been effective in lowering voice pitch, increasing sexual drive, bettering self-esteem, and giving more energy and endurance.

Early Intervention

• Klinefelter syndrome usually is not detected in infancy, but when young boys enter school. The earlier you can make assessment for learning and developmental delays, the sooner intervention can begin, especially for speech-language delays and behavioral difficulties.

• If early intervention is possible in the preschool years, a language-based preschool is recommended.

• Target language processing deficits for school-aged children. Do a complete evaluation, taking into account possible attention deficit disorders. Then you can target language processing.

Curriculum-Based Intervention

- Since the majority of these young men will complete school and have normal life spans, the intervention plan should be curriculum-based and functional. Give students resource assistance. Build a team approach with educators and counselors.

Summary . . . .

Klinefelter syndrome is a chromosomal variation affecting males. Rather than one X and one Y sex chromosome, the affected male will have two, three, or four X chromosomes. Resulting characteristics include sterility, a lack of secondary sex characteristics at puberty, learning disorders, and speech-language deficits. Physical characteristics include tallness, long limbs, underdeveloped genitalia, and enlarged breasts. Self-esteem is generally low, and social development may be delayed.

It's usually difficult to detect Klinefelter syndrome until a child has begun school. But as a speech-language pathologist, start intervention as early as possible with attention to receptive and expressive language skills and articulation. After an evaluation, emphasize language processing. For school-aged boys, a curriculum-based instruction works best.

References • • • • • • • • • • • • • • • • •

Batshaw, M. L. *Children with Disabilities, Fourth Edition.* Baltimore, MD: Paul H. Brookes Publishing Co., 1997.

Gerber, S. E. *Etiology and Prevention of Communicative Disorders, Second Edition.* San Diego, CA: Singular Publishing Group, Inc., 1998.

Gilbert, P. *The A-Z Reference Book of Syndromes and Inherited Disorders, Second Edition.* New York, NY: Chapman & Hall, 1996.

"Klinefelter Syndrome Information." <http://www.genetic.org/ks/aboutxxy.htm> October 27, 1999.

Pore, S. G. & Reed, K. L. *Quick Reference to Speech-Language Pathology.* Gaithersburg, MD: Aspen Publishers, Inc., 1999.

Shprintzen, R. J. *Genetics, Syndromes, and Communication Disorders.* San Diego, CA: Singular Publishing Group, Inc., 1997.

• • • • • • • •

Mental Retardation:
Sotos and Cornelia de Lange Syndromes

This chapter will be a little different from the others because we will look at two syndromes that share common characteristics of mental retardation. There is a documented high correlation of impaired cognition and mental retardation in many syndromes. In this chapter, we will take a closer look at the definitions, characteristics, and speech-language issues of two of these syndromes: Sotos and Cornelia de Lange. Intervention issues will address both syndromes with the primary focus on the cognitive impairment.

There are two national associations specifically concerned with effective practices and advocating for persons with intellectual disabilities: the American Association of Mental Retardation (AAMR, 1999) and the Association for Persons with Severe Handicaps (TASH, 1999). References to the descriptions and missions of these associations are included at the end of this chapter.

Mental retardation is defined by subcategorical levels. *The Diagnostic and Statistical Manual of Mental Disorders, Fourth Edition* (DSM-IV, 1994) definition puts the levels of retardation into the categories designated in the box below.

Those who exhibit cognitive evaluation scores in the range of retardation will present a unique profile, depending on abilities in adaptive functioning, environment, associated complications, and intervention history. Syndromes with a high correlation of mental retardation will show a variance in the level of retardation. Both Sotos syndrome and Cornelia de Lange syndrome are associated with mild, moderate, severe, and profound levels of mental retardation.

IQ Levels of Mental Retardation			
Mild	50-55	to	70
Moderate	35-40	to	50
Severe	20-25	to	35
Profound	below 20-25		

Sotos Syndrome

Syndrome Definition . . . .

Sotos syndrome is a rare, genetic, endocrine condition that causes excessive physical growth during the first years of life. It's primarily a sporadically occurring syndrome, but some autosomal dominant and autosomal recessive forms are seen. A mutation in chromosome #3p21 might be the cause, but etiology is still frequently reported as unknown. Equal numbers of males and females are affected by Sotos syndrome, and only 150 cases are reported worldwide (PEDBASE, 1999). A normal life span can be expected, although monitoring for long-term complications is recommended. This overgrowth syndrome is also known as Cerebral Gigantism syndrome.

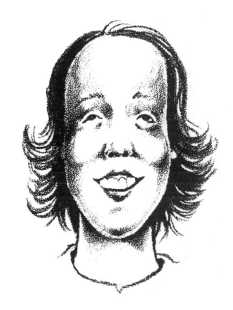

The overgrowth characteristics of Sotos syndrome include excessive stature, advanced bone age, and early maturation (Shprintzen, 1997). These babies are large at birth. Their weight and length are greater than the 90th percentile, and they have abnormally fast growth rates. Diagnosis may be made months or even years following the birth of a child. The extreme rate of growth tends to decelerate in adolescence, and adults generally have large stature but within normal limits.

Respiratory and feeding problems may occur in newborns. Hypotonicity is seen and a poor suck, prolonged drooling, and mouth breathing may all be present. Large hands and feet are commonly found with clumsiness and an awkward gait reported. An increased risk for abdominal tumors may be associated with the syndrome. Seizures are occasionally reported.

Behavioral Characteristics

- delayed motor development

- delayed cognitive development

- poor social adaptation

Characteristics of the face and head are particularly well-defined in Sotos syndrome. A large head with equally large facial features is seen, especially in the mandible, ears, nose, and mouth. The forehead is tall and prominent, the palate is high and arched, the nasal bridge appears flattened, and eyes are downslanted with hypertelorism.

Behavioral Characteristics Profile . . . .

The primary behavioral characteristics associated with Sotos syndrome are explained in the following section.

Delayed Motor Development

Delays in the motor area of development are customary in Sotos syndrome due to the associated hypotonicity. In early life, respiratory and feeding problems are seen, and both gross and fine motor skills are at risk as the child develops. Coordination difficulties may remain into adulthood as clumsiness and an awkward gait are both observed.

Delayed Cognitive Development

Cognitive impairment of varying degrees is reported, and mild-to-moderate levels of retardation are frequent. Specific deficit areas include language learning, mathematics, and socialization. Special education and related services will probably be needed.

Poor Social Adaptation

Children with Sotos syndrome often look older but act younger than their peer groups. They are at-risk for strained interpersonal relationships, can have poor self-esteem, and often present behavioral problems. This gap between appearance and chronological age begins to close in late childhood (Anderson & Buehler, 1999), and it can assist in later social development and skill acquisition. Behavior disturbances that may occur with Sotos syndrome include aggression, irritability, attention deficit disorder, phobias, and obsession.

Speech-Language Issues

- Hypotonia/Speech/ Voice Disorders

- Language Disorders

- Hearing

Speech-Language Issues · · · · · · ·

Here are the specific speech-language issues that SLPs will deal with in clients with Sotos syndrome.

Hypotonia/Speech/Voice Disorders

A marked speech delay is exhibited, and it may be attributed to hypotonicity, developmental delay, or both. Muscle tone may improve with maturity, and speech production will increase in intelligibility. Distortions of phoneme production may be seen and can be connected to dental spacing differences. In the area of voice, a low pitch associated with laryngeal size can be observed. Resonance production is within normal limits.

Language Disorders

A delay in language development for those with Sotos depends on the degree of overall developmental delay and the degree of intellectual impairment. Receptive skills tend to be more highly evolved than expressive language skills. This can cause frustration for the child, and a natural gesture system and/or augmentative communication system may need to be considered.

Hearing

A history of upper respiratory infections and frequent ear infections may be found with Sotos syndrome, but there is not a characteristic hearing loss.

Cornelia de Lange Syndrome

Syndrome Definition . . . .

Cornelia de Lange syndrome appears in most cases to be sporadic or noninherited (Jung, 1989, Batshaw & Perret, 1997), although there is a possibility of autosomal dominant traits in families. The cause is a mutation in either chromosome #3q26.3 or chromosome #17q23. Prevalence is 1/50,000, and males and females are affected in equal numbers.

Cornelia de Lange Syndrome is also known as:

- De Lange syndrome
- Brachman de Lange syndrome

Behavioral Characteristics

- multiple congenital abnormalities/ microcephaly

- severe mental retardation/autistic behavior

- physical features

Behavioral Characteristics Profile . . . .

The primary behavioral characteristics associated with Cornelia de Lange syndrome are explained in the following section.

Multiple Congenital Abnormalities/ Microcephaly

Cornelia de Lange syndrome has been referred to as a dysmorphogenic disorder in which multiple congenital abnormalities are seen (Pore & Reed, 1999). Characteristics include microcephaly, prenatal growth retardation, and short stature with limb anomalies and reductions. Abnormalities of vision such as myopia and nystagmus are observed. Heart malformations, intestinal anomalies, hypotonicity, and seizures are also seen. Early death may occur due to apnea, aspiration, or cardiac complications.

Severe Mental Retardation/Autistic Behavior

Severe mental retardation is exhibited in Cornelia de Lange syndrome, and extensive supports should be expected. Independent living is generally not an option. Self-injurious behaviors and some features associated with autism are seen, particularly in later life. Frequent mood changes and severe temper tantrums may occur.

Physical Features

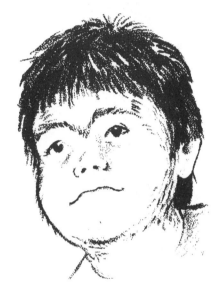

The physical appearance of Cornelia de Lange syndrome is quite distinctive. In addition to the microcephaly, excessive hairiness (hypertrichosis or hirsutism) with a confluent eyebrow (synophrys) and a low anterior hairline are seen. Thick, curled eyelashes are common. A depressed nasal bridge, long philtrum, thin upper lip, and anteverted nostrils are also exhibited.

There are malformations of the ear, which include low set auricles, large pinna size, small external auditory canals, and irregularly slanted outer canals (Jung, 1989). Cleft palate and a lack of facial expression may be noted. Facial features of the syndrome are coarse (Shprintzen, 1997). Micrognathia and Pierre Robin sequence are also possible within Cornelia de Lange syndrome.

Speech-Language Issues . . . .

Severe speech-language deficits are observed in Cornelia de Lange syndrome. Some children do not develop into verbal communicators, and augmentative or alternative communicative means must be considered. Here are some speech language issues for those who develop verbal language.

Speech-Language Delays

The speech-language delays seen in the syndrome are generally severe. The influence of the intellectual disability will play a major part in expectations of language development. Expressive language skills will be more poorly developed than receptive skills, and syntactical development will develop more slowly than vocabulary/ lexicon acquisition. Neurologically-based articulation errors are exhibited with omissions and distortions reported for all phoneme classes.

Voice/Resonance Disorders

Hypernasality is noted in Cornelia de Lange syndrome, and is most likely caused by velopharyngeal insufficiency secondary to the cleft palate. A hoarse voice quality with a low pitch is heard beginning in infancy.

Dysphagia

Children with Cornelia de Lange may experience feeding difficulties and present failure to thrive in their early months. Gastrointestinal disorders associated with reflux and aspiration may be noted, and indications of swallowing abilities must be evaluated. Upper airway obstruction is also common.

Hearing Loss

A conductive hearing loss may be exhibited, and is often secondary to the high number of middle ear difficulties associated with a cleft palate. Approximately 50% of those with Cornelia de Lange exhibit a mild to moderate sensorineural hearing loss (Shprintzen, 1997).

Intervention for syndromes of mental retardation must be guided by the needs of each child. Although levels of retardation were described earlier, each child with an intellectual deficit will exhibit a unique pattern of strength and needs.

Intervention Issues

- Early Intervention

- Team Approach

- Language Therapy

- Augmentative and Alternative Communication

Early Intervention

- In infancy, mental retardation is difficult to diagnose. Children in early intervention and early childhood education are more apt to carry a diagnosis of developmental delay if a definitive diagnosis is not made. Children that present a particular syndrome may be at an advantage with early diagnosis which allows for appropriate programming.

- Provide a communication-rich environment for infants suspected of developmental delays. Strategies can be shared with parents to provide facilitation of communication abilities (Hoge & Parette, 1995).

- Provide services with a transdisciplinary team of "best practice."

- Make early identification of health-related issues and seizures. Multiple medical conditions may be present.

Team Approach

- Speech-language pathologists working with children with intellectual delays should have a team approach that includes various pertinent professionals and the family. Communication disorders are common in syndromes associated with mental retardation, and the speech-language pathologist will play a primary role.

- Audiologists will identify and assess hearing status appropriate for children with retardation. This may mean using test protocol other than pure tone audiometric examination. Tympanometry and sound field testing may be necessary. Monitor hearing status, particularly with recurrent otitis media.

- Occupational therapy will be necessary for children with retardation, and activities of daily living may be an area of concentration.

- Often children with retardation will need physical therapy. Gross motor and fine motor deficits and overall hypotonia can be seen in Sotos and Cornelia de Lange. Those suffering from Sotos syndrome may especially need assistance in additional mobility training.

- A school team can include the professionals mentioned above, special education teachers, and an adapted physical education teacher. A school counselor or psychologist and a job trainer may also be appropriate team members.

Language Therapy

- Needs identified for language therapy in Sotos syndrome include the language that can encourage self-help skills and can assist with successful completion of tasks toward mastery of developmental skills.

- Functional language therapy specifically targets expressive and receptive vocabulary and syntax, and heavily targets pragmatics.

Augmentative and Alternative Communication

- As mental retardation increases in severity, the number of children who will remain nonverbal also increases. Augmentative and alternative communication techniques are appropriate to allow children to become as independent as possible.

- Allowing children to communicate in a multimodal manner is very beneficial. Natural gestures, facial expressions, vocalizations, and body language can be combined with more formal augmentative means to allow children the opportunity to communicate with the people in their environment.

Summary . . . .

Mental retardation is evident in many identified syndromes, and these syndromes also have important speech-language consideration. In this chapter, we've looked at Sotos syndrome and Cornelia de Lange syndrome, two syndromes that are distinguished by various levels of mental retardation.

As a therapist or pathologist, keep in mind that each client who exhibits cognitive evaluation scores in the range of retardation will present an unique profile, and you should treat him/her as an individual. The mental retardation depends on abilities in adaptive functioning, environment, associated complications, and intervention history. Syndromes with a high correlation of mental retardation show this variance in the individualized profiles for each child. Sotos and Cornelia de Lange are associated with mild, moderate, severe, and profound levels of mental retardation.

● ● ● ● ● ● ●

References

"American Association on Mental Retardation. AAMR's mission statement." <http://www.aamr.org/About_AAMR/mission_statement.html> November 9, 1999.

Anderson, R. R. & Buehler, B. A. *What is Sotos Syndrome?* <http://www.well.com/user/sssa/whatisit.htm> November 9, 1999.

Batshaw, M. & Perret, Y. *Children with Disabilities—A Medical Primer, Third Edition.* Baltimore, MD: Paul H. Brookes Publishing Co., 1992.

"Diagnostic and statistical manual of mental disorders, Fourth Edition, DSM-IV." American Psychiatric Association. Washington, DC: 1994.

Gerber, S. E. *Etiology and Prevention of Communicative Disorders, Second Edition.* San Diego, CA: Singular Publishing Group, Inc., 1998.

Gilbert, P. *The A-Z Reference Book of Syndromes and Inherited Disorders, Second Edition.* New York, NY: Chapman & Hall, 1996.

Goodban, M. T. "Survey of Speech and Language Skills with Prognostic Indicators in 116 Patients with Cornelia de Lange Syndrome." *American Journal of Medical Genetics*, Vol. 47, pp. 1059-1063, 1993.

Hoge, D. R. & Parette, H. P. "Facilitating Communicative Development in Young Children with Disabilities." *Infant-Toddler Intervention*, Vol. 5, pp. 113-131, 1995.

Jung, J. *Genetic Syndromes in Communication Disorders.* Austin, Texas: Pro-Ed, 1989.

"National Institute of Neurological Disorders and Stroke (NINDS). Sotos Syndrome." <http://www.healthtouch.com/level1/leaflets/ninds/ninds276.htm> November 9, 1999.

Paul, R. *Language Disorders from Infancy to Adolescence: Assessment and Intervention.* St. Louis, MO: Mosby Year Book, 1995.

"Pediatric Database (PEDBASE). Sotos Syndrome." <http://www.icondata.com/health/pedbase/ tiles/SOTOSYND.HTM> November 9, 1999.

Pore, S. G. & Reed, K. L. *Quick Reference to Speech-Language Pathology.* Gaithersburg, MD: Aspen Publishers, Inc., 1999.

Shprintzen, R. J. *Genetics, Syndromes, and Communication Disorders.* San Diego, CA: Singular Publishing Group, Inc., 1997.

"TASH-Disability Advocacy Worldwide. TASH Homepage." <http://www.tash.org.misc.index.htm> November 9, 1999.

Wetherby, A. M., Warren, S. F., & Reichle, J. (eds.) *Transitions in Prelinguistic Communication.* Baltimore, MD: Paul H. Brookes Publishing Co., 1998.

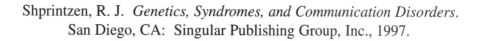

Moebius Syndrome

Characteristics

- Early feeding and swallowing difficulties
- Articulation impairment
- Expressive language impairment
- Vision difficulties

- little or no facial movement

- affects males and females equally

- some consider it a *sequence* rather than a *syndrome*

- caused by underdeveloped facial-cranial nerves

- weak articulation and expressive language

Syndrome Definition . . . .

Moebius syndrome is considered a rare condition. It is recognized at birth by a baby's lack of facial movement. Males and females are equally affected. The cause of the syndrome is a subject of debate among professionals. Some think it's due to spontaneous mutation, while others think an autosomal dominant inheritance is responsible. A third possibility is the presence of illness, drug abuse, or accident in the mother during the first three months of pregnancy.

Shprintzen (1997) argues that Moebius is not a syndrome at all, but a sequence disorder. He states that not all multiple-anomaly disorders are actually syndromes. A *syndrome* is defined as multiple anomalies present in a child having a single primary cause. A *sequence* is a disorder in which the multiple anomalies present in a child are actually secondary disorders. A single anomaly which occurs during embryonic development sets off a chain of reactions which cause multiple changes. Therefore, "a sequence is the presence of multiple anomalies in an individual where most or all of the anomalies present are caused secondarily by a single known or presumed structural anomaly or error in development."

Whether we classify Moebius as a syndrome or sequence, the presumed cause of the multiple anomalies is a failure of development in specific blood vessels at a critical stage in utero. The main effect is exhibited in the baby's face. Little expression or movement is ever seen in the face and the baby's eyes and

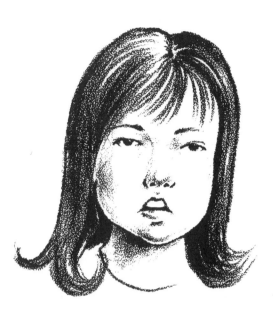

mouth remain open most of the time. The facial muscles are supplied by specific cranial nerves originating in the brainstem. Studies suggest that these nerves are small and underdeveloped.

Weakness is also present in the tongue and palate muscles. Mandibular deficiency (shortening) is also caused by the vascular disruption during embryonic development. All of these structures are involved in sucking and swallowing movements, resulting in extreme feeding difficulty for the infant. Tube feeding is sometimes necessary to insure adequate nutrition for growth. Aspiration of milk, saliva, and mucus are serious threats in a young infant and can lead to pneumonia. As the baby matures, many of these problems improve, although clearing the oral cavity remains a challenge for the toddler. It's not unusual for solid food to become lodged in the cheeks of a child due to difficulty with facial and oral muscles.

The primary speech difficulties evidenced are in articulation and expressive language. Weak facial and oral muscles make coordinated, controlled movement of the lips and tongue very difficult. Resonance can also be somewhat muffled due to muscular weakness. Voice, hearing, and receptive language are usually within normal limits.

Lack of muscle control in closing the eyes can lead to additional problems. Minute particles of dust can settle and remain on a child's cornea because they are not washed away by normal protective blinking. The eyes must be monitored closely for scratches or ulcerations of the cornea.

Additional limb anomalies that can occur include abnormalities in the finger size and club foot (35% of cases). Weakness in the chest muscles may also occur.

The behavioral characteristics associated with Moebius syndrome are explained in the following section.

Early Feeding & Swallowing Difficulties

Feeding problems immediately following birth are the most acute issue in the syndrome. Tube feeding is often necessary in the early months to prevent aspiration of milk and to avoid exhaustion in the infant. Weak oral-facial muscles mean the baby has to work very hard to accomplish intake of expected amounts of milk compared to typical babies.

Although facial muscles will never achieve normal muscle tone, the child will gradually learn to develop adequate feeding and swallowing skills. However, it's not unusual for a child to experience residual sucking problems. Aspiration and choking continue to be threats in toddlers. Food can easily become lodged in the cheeks or mouth cavities due to poor muscle control. Preschool children with Moebius should be monitored carefully at snack and meal times until feeding patterns are consistently accurate.

Articulation Impairment

Accurate formation of the phonemes for language requires coordinated oral-facial muscle movement. The muscle weakness resulting from the syndrome creates difficulty in precise articulatory movement. A delay in acquisition of consonants and vowels due to weak musculature results in a child who is difficult to understand. Poor muscle movement also adds to resonance and vocal quality deviations.

Expressive Language Impairment

Since production of sounds is difficult, children tend to use short phrases and abbreviated utterances to express their needs. Consequently, development of expressive output of language becomes deviant or slow to develop. Messages may be telegraphic in nature or they may lack important production qualities to insure accurate transference of the idea or thought. Interaction with others may be a source of frustration due to difficulty expressing needs and desires. Expressive production of language must be encouraged and stimulated to prevent more significant deficits in academic learning.

Vision Difficulties

Infants are at risk for infection and damage because they can't close their eyes. Parents and teachers should watch for any redness or excessive watering in a young child's eyes. Any complaints of pain or discomfort should be investigated. Early treatment for any abrasions to the cornea could prevent later scarring or other permanent damage.

Speech-Language Issues . . . .

The speech-language pathologist should be aware of several specific aspects of the communication profile in Moebius syndrome. These aspects are summarized in the following information.

Articulation

Intelligible speech can be significantly compromised during early development without speech-language therapy for sound production. Teach parents and teachers techniques to stimulate accurate sound production skills. Lips and tongue muscles are critical for accurate production of consonant and vowel sounds. Use exercises to strengthen oral-motor movement and specific tongue and lip positions. Muscle strength deficits can affect vocal quality aspects of speech production such as nasal resonance and clarity of tone. These aspects of speech production should also be monitored and addressed as necessary.

Speech-Language Issues

• Articulation

• Expressive Language

• Feeding and Swallowing

Expressive Language

Receptive understanding of language should be approximately age-commensurate. It will be important to carefully monitor and stimulate all aspects of verbal language due to muscle weaknesses that can affect output development. Oral-motor exercises and articulation aspects will be primary areas of focus, but encourage children with the syndrome to expand utterances and practice using expressive language consistently. Look carefully for semantic vocabulary terms, concepts, syntactic structures, and pragmatic aspects of verbal language in conjunction with developmental milestones.

Feeding and Swallowing

Feeding difficulties are often present during the early months of life due to poor muscle control. This causes a weak sucking response, compromising the oral preparatory phase for feeding and swallowing. You will be involved almost immediately to address pediatric swallowing issues and to assist in feeding procedures to ensure adequate nutrition. While musculature will gradually improve, stages of chewing and swallowing should be carefully monitored throughout the preschool years due to aspiration and choking tendencies.

Intervention Issues . . . .

The speech-language issues in Moebius syndrome are relatively mild compared to many of the other syndromes evidenced in the preschool years. Most difficulties originate from facial and oral-motor muscle weakness. Prognosis is fairly good, and most deficits can be remediated to a functional, independent level.

Articulation

• Stimulate and directly target acquisition of sounds

during preschool years. A motor approach might be most successful due to poor muscle control.

- Oral air pressure for sound production may be compromised by weak oral musculature. Balanced resonance may also be compromised, requiring exercises to strengthen velopharyngeal valving.

- Initiate oral-motor exercises to strengthen range and strength of movement in the oral articulators, particularly coordinated tongue and lip movements.

Expressive Language

- Expressive output may be abbreviated because of muscular problems and weakness of speech production. Length of utterance should be gradually increased as muscle strength and articulation improve.

- Stimulate expressive language during the preschool years to circumvent later delays. Monitor all aspects of language development to ensure compliance with developmental norms.

Feeding and Swallowing

- Evaluate and monitor feeding and swallowing capabilities from birth through the preschool years or until the problem resolves.

- Modifications and compensations may be necessary until the child masters the sucking response and oral-muscle control at a functional level.

- Parents and teachers may need specific training to become comfortable with feeding and swallowing techniques.

Team Approach

- An ophthamologist may need to monitor cornea damage or eye difficulties in early years due to poor muscle control.

- Physical and occupational therapy consultations might assist in ideas to strengthen oral-motor skills.

Summary

Moebius syndrome is primarily characterized by weak facial and oral muscles resulting in little facial movement or expression. An open-eyes-and-mouth posture is typical in infants. There is some debate regarding the cause, but most agree that the syndrome originates from an interruption during development of the cranial nerves in the oral-facial area. This occurs in the first three months of embryonic development. Immediate concerns focus on feeding and swallowing issues and gradually evolve to speech-language production issues. Limb malformation, particularly fingers, is also possible.

Moebius is considered rare. It affects both females and males equally. The characteristics are not life-threatening, and residual effects are fairly minimal. Once the early years are weathered and interventions (e.g., improving muscle movement to improve speech production) have addressed deficits, life expectancy and prognosis are relatively normal. Features don't exclude children from any activities.

Surgical intervention continues to improve prognosis for those with Moebius syndrome. The media have profiled surgeons who provide these children with a "smile." Despite the rarity of the condition, publicity generated by emotional appeal is resulting in significant medical progress.

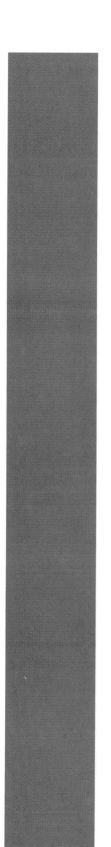

References

Gilbert, P. *The A-Z Reference Book of Syndromes and Inherited Disorders, Second Edition.* New York, NY: Chapman & Hall, 1996.

Shprintzen, R. J. *Genetics, Syndromes, and Communication Disorders.* San Diego, CA: Singular Publishing Group, Inc., 1997.

The Mucopolysaccharidoses (MPS)

Characteristics

- Developmental delay
- Cognitive impairment
- Behavior problems

- a series of 6-10 syndromes

- features include short stature, hirsutism, bushy eyebrows

- 1/16,000 to 1/216,000 live births

- no cure

- wide spectrum of clinical severity

Syndrome Definition . . . .

The mucopolysaccharidoses (or the MPS) are rare, metabolic, hereditary diseases that result in connective tissue deformities. Those affected by these diseases are unable to produce enzymes that break down fats and carbohydrates in the body causing the excesses to be stored in various body tissues and organs. Accumulations of acids are also stored in the central nervous system and in the peripheral tissues and joints.

The mucopolysaccharidoses are chronic, progressive, and display a wide spectrum of clinical severity. The disorders are generally numbered MPS I-VII, depending on how the diseases exhibit and based on the degree of excessive mucopolysaccharide being stored. The wide clinical variability depends on the enzyme deficiency. Some characteristics found in most of the mucopolysaccaridoses include:

- clinical features not always apparent at birth
- progressive mental retardation
- orthopedic problems/short stature
- characteristic physical appearance

Some types of mucopolysaccharidoses lead to progressive mental retardation, and others are potentially fatal. There is currently no cure for the mucopolysaccharidoses, and historically there has been no successful direct treatment (Brown, 1999).

There are six to ten different mucopolysaccharidoses, based on how they are described and combined. Many of the mucopolysaccharidoses have subtypes separated by severity and age of onset.

The mucopolysaccharidoses can be tested for via amniocentesis prior to birth, and skeletal x-rays and urine analysis are common in postnatal periods. All forms of mucopolysaccharidoses (other than Hunter syndrome) are inherited, autosomal recessive, and have a 25% risk for recurrence. The affected chromosome number varies with the type of mucopolysaccharidoses.

The Mucopolysaccharidoses

MPS I-H	Hurler Syndrome
MPS I-S	Scheie Syndrome
MPS I-H/S	Hurler-Scheie Compound
MPS II	Hunter Syndrome
MPS III (or MPS V)	Sanfilippo Syndrome
MPS IV	Morquio Syndrome
MPS VI	Maroteaux-Lamy Syndrome
MPS VII	Sly Syndrome

Hunter syndrome was the first mucopolysaccharidosis discovered in 1917. Hurler syndrome was identified shortly after, in 1919. These two syndromes were primarily noted for their coarse facial features and skeletal anomalies. Morquio syndrome was identified in 1929, and in 1952, Brante suggested the term "Mucopolysaccharidoses" as a storage disease (PEDBASE, 1998). The remaining mucopolysaccharidoses were identified in the following order: Scheie (1962), Sanfilippo (1963), and Maroteaux-Lamy (1963). Incidence numbers for all six range from 1/16,000 to 1/216,000 live births (Brown, 1999; Gerber, 1998).

The clinical features of the mucopolysaccharidoses are not usually apparent at birth. As the child moves through infancy and childhood, short stature, hirsutism, and atypical development become apparent. Thick lips, a flat nasal bridge, an open-mouth position, and coarse facial features may also help diagnose MPS. Coarse, unruly hair and bushy eyebrows are also noted. Skeletal x-rays and urine tests may be used for diagnosis of mucopolysaccharidoses in young children.

Behavioral Characteristics Profile . . . .

Although the mucopolysaccharidoses are distinct, there are general behavior characteristics that are observed in all of them. We will review the general characteristics in this section, then look at each mucopolysaccharidosis separately.

- Developmental Delay
- Cognitive Impairment
- Behavior Problems

Developmental Delay

The symptoms may not be apparent at birth, but progressive involvement soon becomes evident. Degeneration of both mental and physical abilities are discernable as the child ages. Visual deficits, particularly clouding of the cornea, are noted. Joint and skeletal disorders, including stiffness, contractures, kyphosis, and carpal tunnel syndrome are seen. Facial features become coarser with age. Impaired hearing involvement and shortness of stature occur with development. Heart and internal organ complications may also occur.

Cognitive Impairment

Mild-to-severe cognitive impairment is evident in the mucopolysaccharidoses. Hunter syndrome, in the milder version, and Maroteaux-Lamy syndrome show the least amount of cognitive impairment, while Sly syndrome and Sanfilippo syndrome manifest more severe cognitive impairments. The deterioration of mental abilities appears to be progressive.

Behavior Problems

There is a high incidence of certain behavior problems present in all of the mucopolysaccharidoses. Hurler and Hunter syndromes may cause children to be anxious or fearful, and sleep problems are also frequent. Hyperactivity is apparent at various periods in the development of syndrome characteristics, and other behavior problems such as aggression or defiance may evolve.

Sanfilippo syndrome seems to cause the most severe behavior problems among the group. The problems are restlessness, aggression, and destructiveness, and these behaviors directed toward siblings and parents can be catastrophic for the family.

Let's now take a look at the six mucopolysaccharidoses and their variations in greater detail.

MPS I-H: Hurler Syndrome

Hurler syndrome is a severe form of mucopolysaccaridoses, and usually results in the person's death either before age ten or in the second decade of life. The most likely cause of death is heart failure, pneumonia, or another severe respiratory tract infection.

Clients who have mucopolysaccharidoses may appear to be asymptomatic at birth, but develop more identifiable clinical features with age. Growth failure after infancy is apparent, as is a progressive coarsening of facial features. Clouding of the corneas, repeated upper-respiratory infections, and chronic nasal discharge are common. Enlargement of the liver and spleen and inguinal hernias are also seen. A skeletal deformity (claw hand deformity) evolves as spasticity develops and joint immobility progresses.

Hurler
Syndrome

Communication disorder issues include the possibility of mild-to-moderate sensorineural hearing loss, and some conductive components due to otitis media and upper respiratory infections. Small, misaligned teeth and an enlarged tongue have been exhibited and can be the cause of faulty articulation production. Progressive mental retardation is evidenced, and microcephaly has been noted. Expect language disorders to correspond to the cognitive impairment.

MPS I-S: Scheie Syndrome

Scheie syndrome may also be referred to as MPS V rather than MPS I-S (Batshaw, 1997). Scheie syndrome is difficult to identify prior to age six, and is milder than Hurler syndrome. Stiff joints and corneal clouding are noted in Scheie syndrome, but normal intelligence and a typical life span can be expected. Hearing loss may be associated, but it is not severe.

MPS II: Hunter Syndrome

Hunter syndrome is the only MPS to have an X-linked inheritance pattern, which means it occurs almost exclusively in males. It's seen primarily in those of European descent. It is similar to Hurler syndrome, although there is no corneal clouding and there is greater variability seen in onset and severity.

There are two types of Hunter syndrome: one is severe and the other is mild. The milder form allows patients to survive to adulthood, and the cognitive impairment is mild or absent. The more severe form causes death prior to age fifteen. Severe mental retardation, hyperactivity, and aggressiveness are all noted in Hunter syndrome.

A decrease of overall body growth is seen between ages two and six, and dwarfism is common. An enlarged head, skeletal anomalies, abdominal hernias, and heart disease are all seen in Hunter syndrome. The distinctive coarse facial features of the MPS appear, and chronic upper and lower respiratory tract infections are common. Noisy breathing, narrow nasal passages, and large adenoids are observed.

A hearing impairment may appear by age three, but will not typically be severe. The loss may be conductive, sensorineural, or mixed. Anomalies of the round window and middle ear have been noted. The child with Hunter syndrome may also have reduced vestibular function.

MPS III: Sanfilippo Syndrome

There are four distinct types of Sanfilippo syndrome caused by four different enzyme defects, but the four types are clinically similar enough to be included in one MPS. The general characteristics include mild coarsening of features, joint stiffness, and progressive mental retardation in all types. Other characteristics include mild somatic changes, severe central nervous system effects, seizures, and progressive dementia (Jung, 1989; Batshaw, 1997).

Identification usually occurs between ages two and six, and severe behavior disturbances are noted. Hyperactivity, aggression, poor sleep patterns, temper tantrums, and destructive behaviors are all exhibited during this time. Mild enlargement of the liver is also evident, as is chronic diarrhea in 50% of the population (Brown, 1999; Batshaw, 1997). Progressive spasticity and ataxia are obvious, and these will affect ambulation and feeding. In the most severe form (MPS IIIA), death occurs between ten and twenty.

There is no apparent hearing loss associated with Sanfilippo syndrome as in the other mucopolysaccharidoses. Communication instruction is valuable for the social aspects of language as the behavior disorders emerge. When cognition begins to fail and dementia develops, use language therapy aggressively.

MPS IV: Morquio Syndrome

Morquio syndrome is most identifiable by a dwarfism caused by severe abnormal bone development. As with the other mucopolysaccharidoses, those with Morquio syndrome appear normal at birth and the characteristics become more apparent in infancy and childhood. Three types of Morquio syndrome have been identified and each differs in the severity of symptoms and by the age at which the syndrome is detected.

Shortened stature and difficulties with continence are common in the most severe form of the disorder. Mental development is generally unaffected. Life expectancy is 30 or 40 years, and the cause of death is most likely due to cardiopulmonary complications. The intermediate form presents the expected characteristics in a less severe form, and it is identifiable in childhood. The mild form of the disorder presents with nearly normal stature and mild skeletal anomalies, and is diagnosed during late childhood or adolescence.

Communication concerns in Morquio syndrome center on skeletal changes that may affect dentition and articulation. Pathologies of the middle ear are associated. Chronic or recurrent otitis media was found in nearly 80% of the population in one study, and a mixed or sensorineural hearing loss can manifest itself by approximately age 10 (Jung, 1989).

MPS VI: Maroteaux-Lamy Syndrome

Expect intact intelligence in Maroteaux-Lamy syndrome. Pronounced skeletal deformities with curvature of the spine and restricted joint mobility are seen. A large head, a short neck, and a broad flat nose with large nostrils are also exhibited. Skin and hair are thick and coarse, and short stature is common. Jung (1989) noted that the clinical features of MPS VI closely resemble those of Hurler syndrome, except that in Maroteaux-Lamy, intelligence is normal.

There are two types of Maroteaux-Lamy, one mild and one more severe. Conductive hearing impairment due to chronic otitis media is evident in the more severe type.

MPS VII: Sly Syndrome

Sly syndrome has an enormous impact on cognitive and communication skills and orthopedic development. It's a rare type of mucopolysaccharidoses with age of onset determining the severity of the syndrome. Life expectancy is from ten to twenty years. Failure to thrive, pneumonia, and corneal clouding are evident as the child ages. Decreased joint mobility, short stature, and characteristic facial features are also evident. A neonatal form of Sly syndrome can result in infant death (Brown, 1999). Mild to profound mental retardation is seen in Sly syndrome, accompanied by developmental delays in speech and language development.

Speech-Language Issues . . . .

There are some speech-language issues that apply for all the MPS. Communication skills will vary greatly. As cognitive skills and skeletal structure show progressive deterioration, you need to carefully monitor needs. Accurate evaluation and assessment of speech-language and hearing abilities may be jeopardized by the decrease in motor and intellectual skills.

Hearing Impairment

The possibility of hearing impairment is prominent in each MPS. A wide range in type and degree of hearing impairment exists. Hearing impairments will generally be progressive, so long-term management will be needed.

Language Impairment

Language skills will vary widely within the MPS and will parallel cognitive skills. Typical language developmental milestones may be met, but as symptoms of the MPS become more apparent, language skills may be lost. In Sanfilippo, Hurler, and Sly syndromes, severe retardation will profoundly affect language usage, and you may consider augmentative communication.

Dementia

Progressive dementia has specifically been identified in Sanfilippo syndrome. This means that cognitive and language skills will decline as the symptoms become manifested.

Articulation/Speech Production

One of the major characteristics in all the mucopolysaccharidoses is the severity of orthopedic changes due to acid accumulation in the joints. The skeletal and joint changes can affect the skull and facial skeleton. Articulation production depends on precise and accurate movement patterns. These patterns may be jeopardized by stiffness and contracture of joints.

The facial features associated with the MPS may interfere with speech production. The structure of the nasal passages and nose, thick lips, and open-mouth position all affect articulation.

Most children with mucopolysaccharidoses need special education and related services as they progress through the symptoms of the disease. Specific intervention issues for these children follow.

Early Intervention

- Early intervention is recommended, but it's often difficult to begin due to the late manifestation of many of the symptoms of the mucopolysaccharidoses.

- If an early diagnosis *is* possible, intervention services can be put into place to reduce the effect of the degeneration. Maximize intellectual gain with early stimulation prior to deterioration.

Hearing Status

- Expect hearing impairment in any of the mucopolysaccharidoses. Due to the variance in type and degree of loss, no single approach to management is best.

- Early, accurate evaluation and continual, long-term monitoring are essential. These may sound basic, but can be challenging in this population with its associated motor and cognitive deficits.

Evaluation and Assessment

- Accurate evaluation and assessment of overall skills (particularly in the areas of speech and language) may be difficult due to reduced motor skills and cognition. Once again, early diagnosis and a team approach are imperative to maintaining communication skills whenever possible.

Alternative and Augmentative Communication

- With the progressive loss of skills common to the mucopolysaccharidoses, the patient may become a candidate for using an alternative or augmentative communication strategy.

- Signing may *not* be the best choice for many affected by MPS due to skeletal, joint, and hand deformities (e.g., carpal tunnel syndrome). Adaptive signs are certainly acceptable.

- If you use a visual device, assess the client's visual abilities carefully and make sure you choose the device based on motor ability.

- Multimodal communication may be a good idea with a combination of verbal, nonverbal, and augmentative techniques to capitalize on all communication options.

- An occupational therapist and physical therapist can assist the SLP in making positioning suggestions for optimal use of devices.

Life span Planning

- Many people suffering from the MPS have life span expectations well below average—some will not outlive childhood. Communication skills for these clients should concentrate on the present. Allow these clients the full extent of functional use possible.

- Children with Scheie, Morquio, Maroteaux-Lamy, and the milder type of Hunter syndrome may retain typical or mildly-impaired cognition and have longer life expectancies.

Team Approach

- Support and assistance from a variety of team members are essential for the child with the MPS because of the regression in skills and behavior.

- Medical professionals including neurologists, orthopedic specialists, otorhinolaryngologists, gastrointestinal doctors, opthalmologists, and cardiovascular specialists are all possible team members.

- Audiologists will play a primary role on the team due to the progressive hearing impairment found in the population. Because the type and severity of impairment will vary, the audiologist's role will include continual monitoring of hearing status.

- As an SLP, you can play an important role in several areas. Provision of language therapies may be a primary role, depending on lost language skills. You should become familiar with the proper language treatment for clients with dementia. Articulation therapy and monitoring of hearing will also be important areas to address.

- Genetic counseling may be necessary due to the hereditary nature of mucopolysaccharidoses.

- Involve psychologists as life expectancy issues and disabling conditions develop. Known behavior difficulties can also be attended to with psychological referral.

- As always, include families on the treatment team. Having a child who has been diagnosed with a life-threatening condition and who has lost abilities can be catastrophic for families. They will need team support and assistance as they care for their child.

Summary . . . .

The mucopolysaccharidoses are a group of rare, hereditary, metabolic diseases that cause anomalies and deformities related to the connective tissues of the body. They are chronic and progressive and can display an extensive spectrum of clinical severity. This wide clinical variability depends on the enzyme deficiency. Those who are affected by these diseases are unable to produce enzymes that break down fats and carbohydrates in the body. The excesses are then stored in various body tissues and organs. Accumulations of the acids are stored in the grey and white matter of the central nervous system and in the peripheral tissues and joints.

There are between six and ten different mucopolysaccharidoses based on how they are described and combined. Many of the specific mucopolysaccharidoses have subtypes delineated relative to severity and age of onset. The disorders are referred to as MPS I-VII, depending on which of the characteristics are exhibited and the degree of excessive mucopolysaccharide being stored. In review, the specified types of mucopolysaccharidoses are:

MPS I-H	Hurler Syndrome
MPS I-S	Scheie Syndrome

MPS I H/S	Hurler-Scheie Compound
MPS II	Hunter Syndrome
MPS III (or MPS V)	Sanfilippo Syndrome
MPS IV	Morquio Syndrome
MPS VI	Maroteaux-Lamy Syndrome
MPS VII	Sly Syndrome

Each disorder has its own characteristics in addition to the general ones they all share. Accurate diagnosis and early intervention are imperative in providing services to children with mucopolysaccharidoses, and a team approach for support and treatment is highly recommended.

●   ●   ●   ●   ●   ●   ●

References

Batshaw, M. L. *Children with Disabilities, Fourth Edition.* Baltimore, MD: Paul H. Brookes Publishing Co., 1997.

Batshaw, M. & Perret, Y. *Children with Disabilities-A Medical Primer, Third Edition.* Baltimore, MD: Paul H. Brookes Publishing Co., 1992.

Brown, M. B. *Handbook of Neurodevelopmental and Genetic Disorders in Children.* New York, NY: The Guilford Press, 1999.

Gerber, S. E. *Etiology and Prevention of Communicative Disorders, Second Edition.* San Diego, CA: Singular Publishing Group, Inc., 1998.

Gilbert, P. *The A-Z Reference Book of Syndromes and Inherited Disorders, Second Edition.* New York, NY: Chapman & Hall, 1996.

Jung, J. *Genetic Syndromes in Communication Disorders.* Austin, Texas: Pro-Ed, 1989.

"Mucopolysaccharidosis information from Merck Manual." <http://merck.com/!!vALonlpe&vALtH3WAf/peds/mmanual/html/znikjeehi.htm> July 15, 1998.

"Mucopolysaccharidosis information." <http://www.icondata.com/health/pedbase/files/MUCOPOLY.HTM> July 18, 1998.

"Pediatric Database (PEDBASE)." <http://www.icondata. com/health/pedbase/ tiles/.HTM> November 9, 1999.

Shprintzen, R. J. *Genetics, Syndromes, and Communication Disorders.* San Diego, CA: Singular Publishing Group, Inc., 1997.

Notes . . . .

Noonan Syndrome

Characteristics

- Cognitive impairment
- Motor delays
- Early feeding and swallowing difficulties
- Articulation impairment
- Hearing loss
- Vision impairment

- congenital heart defects

- short stature

- unusual facial characteristics

- 1/1,000 to 1/2,500

- features vary, making diagnosis difficult

Syndrome Definition . . . .

In 1963, pediatric cardiologist Dr. Jacqueline Noonan reported on a close association between a specific congenital heart defect, short stature, and unusual facial features. These three main features were variable in degree of severity in children, but appeared to be consistently present in a group.

- **Congenital heart defects** can be diagnosed at birth. The range of heart defects vary in severity from those that need no treatment to those that require medication or cardiac surgical intervention. The heart defects can be one or more of the following cardiac problems.

    a. Pulmonary stenosis occurs when a valve in the pulmonary artery is narrow or poorly formed. This is the most common heart defect in Noonan syndrome.

    b. Atrial septal defect occurs in the wall between the two upper chambers of the heart.

    c. Ventricular septal defect occurs in the wall of the heart between the two ventricles.

- **Short stature** typically puts children in the lower 10th percentile of the growth range. The short stature is not as extreme as in other syndromes (e.g., Turner's syndrome), and body proportions in Noonan syndrome are appropriate.

- The presence of **unusual facial characteristics** are distinct but become less noticeable as the child matures. Some of the facial characteristics include the following:

    a. The eyes are widely spaced, tend to slant downward, and the eyelids are frequently droopy. These characteristics persist throughout life.

    b. The neck has a webbed appearance due to a loose fold of skin in the nape (like Turner's syndrome) and exacerbated by a short neck length and low hairline.

    c. The ears tend to be set low on the head and have distinctive lobes that bend forward.

    d. The bridge of the nose frequently has a flattened appearance.

Additional characteristics may include cleft palate (often submucous), hearing loss, vision deficits, and initial feeding problems. The actual features present vary from individual to individual, making diagnosis difficult. For example, facial features noted at birth may change through the adult years. Other clients may not evidence any of the common facial features, resulting in a missed diagnosis.

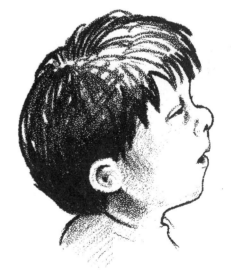

The cause of Noonan syndrome is unknown, but inheritance appears to be genetic by autosomal dominant transference. Incidence is reported to range from 1/1,000 to 1/2,500 (Batshaw & Perret, 1992; Gilbert, 1996). Both genders can be affected. Males tend to have small genitals and undescended testes, which may require surgery in the preschool years. Females tend to resemble those with Turner's syndrome and there is thought to be a close genetic association because of many shared characteristics.

The behavioral characteristics associated with Noonan syndrome are explained in the following section.

Cognitive Impairment

Intelligence levels range from normal to learning disabilities and/or mild mental retardation. Cognitive deficits are perceived during the preschool years due to delays in development. Children tend to mature later and play with younger children, resulting in lower-level skills during the acquisition period.

Motor Delays

Delays are noted in development of motor skills during the preschool years due to poor muscle control. Perceptual motor abnormalities are also apparent, especially in vision. Developmental milestones are delayed, but usually not significantly discrepant beyond the first few years.

Early Feeding & Swallowing Difficulties

Poor muscle strength and control are first evidenced in a weak suck response. Children often have difficulty with feeding and swallowing in the infant stage of development. The difficulties usually resolve in the first few months to a year, but they may require modification and intervention immediately following birth. Extreme cases may require a feeding tube to insure nutritional intake until maturation and intervention begin to resolve the problems. Vomiting can also be an aspect of these difficulties.

Articulation Impairment

Children with Noonan often demonstrate delays in sound acquisition. The articulation deficits are secondary to several of the features characteristic to Noonan syndrome, like cleft palate, hearing loss, poor muscle control, and possible cognitive impairments. The deficits can also carry into vocal aspects of sound production such as nasal resonance and vocal quality.

Hearing Loss

Clients can demonstrate a sensorineural hearing loss, conductive loss, or a mix of the two. The loss tends to correlate with the clefting aspects of Noonan syndrome, but structural deficits in ear formation can also affect internal structural development. Middle ear drainage via the Eustachian tube can be compromised during the preschool years, resulting in frequent ear infections or otitis media.

Vision Impairment

Some children demonstrate difficulties in vision, specifically a squint or myopia (nearsightedness). Deficits may be subtle and missed until placed in an educational setting. Visual deficits can usually be treated with corrective glasses and do not significantly impair the child.

Speech-Language Issues . . . .

Speech-Language Issues

- Articulation

- Voice

- Feeding & Swallowing

- Hearing

- Language

As an SLP, you should be aware of several specific aspects of the communication profile in Noonan syndrome. These aspects are summarized in the following information.

Articulation

Deficits in articulation are secondary to some of the facial features. For example, a malocclusion present due to cleft palate could cause potential problems with sound production skills. A hearing loss could also impact articulation development.

Voice

Problems in voice production are also secondary to primary features. If a cleft is present, hypernasality is possible. Occasionally, the vocal quality will also be hoarse, which is secondary to poor muscle control or structural deviations. Projectile vomiting, occurring consistently through the early years, could also contribute to hoarseness. The consistent regurgitation of acid over the vocal folds can compromise a clear vocal quality. However, once the vomiting is resolved, vocal quality will often resume a clear quality over time.

Feeding & Swallowing

Feeding difficulties are often present during the early months due to poor muscle control. This causes a weak sucking response which compromises the oral preparatory phase for feeding and swallowing. Vomiting can also be associated with this aspect, usually of a projectile nature. However, the feeding and swallowing problems generally resolve during the first year.

Hearing

In some cases, a sensorineural hearing loss and/or conductive impairment occurs. If associated structural problems of clefting are present, otitis media is also a good possibility and can cause conductive hearing loss.

Language

Language acquisition will be primarily impacted by any cognitive impairment which may be part of the syndrome. Pragmatic social language can also be impaired due to self-consciousness regarding facial features, slow maturity, and general developmental delays.

Intervention Issues

- Articulation
- Voice
- Hearing
- Language
- Feeding & Swallowing
- Team Approach

Intervention Issues . . . .

Although the speech-language issues in Noonan syndrome appear fairly extensive, the severity of impairments is milder than in many syndromes. This means less intensive and long-term therapeutic services. Prognosis is fairly good and most of the deficits can be remediated to a functional, independent level.

Articulation

- Stimulate and directly target acquisition of sounds during preschool years.

- Use an oral-motor approach due to poor muscle control.

- Oral air pressure for sound production may be compromised by a submucous cleft. This should be monitored and appropriate modifications implemented to compensate for structural deficits.

- Orthodontia may be necessary to assist articulation positioning if malocclusions are present.

Voice

- If hypernasality is present, check for submucous cleft. Use prosthetic devices or exercises to strengthen intraoral air pressure to accomplish appropriate oral-nasal resonance.

- Vocal quality should be monitored if hoarseness is present. Introduce good vocal hygiene habits and frequent hydration, especially if projectile vomiting is part of the syndrome.

Hearing

- Hearing acuity should be monitored on a regular basis to check for otitis media or fluctuating conductive loss.

- Hearing aids or compensatory strategies, such as amplification and speech reading, should be used to supplement for hearing loss.

Language

- Language acquisition will be delayed, consistent with cognitive abilities. Receptive and expressive language development should be stimulated intensively during the preschool years to circumvent compounded language deficits.

- Pragmatic language may need to be specifically addressed to build confidence in social skills. Rules for interaction with age peers should be introduced in carryover situations to increase appropriate language interaction.

Feeding & Swallowing

- Feeding and swallowing capabilities should be evaluated and monitored from birth through the first year, or until the problem has resolved.

- Modifications and compensations may be necessary until the sucking response and oral muscle control has been mastered to a functional level.

- Parents may need specific training to become comfortable with techniques used in the home setting.

Team Approach

- A pediatric cardiologist will need to monitor the congenital heart defects on a regular basis. Medication or surgery might be necessary in a small number of children.

- A pediatrician will need to monitor growth throughout childhood.

- An ophthamologist may need to be involved if squint or myopia (nearsightedness) is present. Vision deficits can usually be corrected by glasses.

- Physical therapy and occupational therapy consultation may be necessary to intervene on "clumsiness" resulting from poor muscle control and general motor delays.

- A teacher specializing in learning disabilities may be necessary in the educational setting, especially in the early childhood years, because of the child's late development. Splintered academic skills are likely to be demonstrated during the early elementary years.

Summary

Noonan syndrome is diagnosed when a pattern of physical characteristics accompanies specific congenital heart defects. The associated physical characteristics are the prime factors in diagnosis. Many of the features of the syndrome are found in the general population, but when a number of them occur together, Noonan should be considered as a possible diagnosis. Specific features (in addition to heart defects diagnosed at birth) include short stature, facial features of widely-spaced eyes with a downward slant, webbed neck, low-set ears with lobes bent forward, and flattened bridge of the nose. Additional features can include cleft palate, hearing loss, mild cognitive impairments, and small genitals in males.

Children with the syndrome usually lead very normal lives. In some cases, heart defects will require surgical intervention, but most simply are monitored or controlled with medication. The short stature is not extreme and it's more irritating than problematic for the client. Facial features tend to modify with maturity and become less noticeable over time. Many adults with Noonan are never diagnosed due to manageability of symptoms and relatively normal function in the school setting with intervention during the early years. The preschool years are very important for focused intervention because most of the characteristics can be resolved. Special services should be minimal beyond elementary school education.

References

Batshaw, M. & Perret, Y. *Children with Disabilities—A Medical Primer, Third Edition*. Baltimore, MD: Paul H. Brookes Publishing Co., 1992.

Gilbert, P. *The A-Z Reference Book of Syndromes and Inherited Disorders, Second Edition*. New York, NY: Chapman & Hall, 1996.

Shprintzen, R. J. *Genetics, Syndromes, and Communication Disorders*. San Diego, CA: Singular Publishing Group, Inc., 1997.

Notes •

Pierre Robin Sequence

Characteristics

- Persistent apnea
- Central nervous system impairment
- Mental retardation

- underdeveloped jaw

- displaced tongue

- breathing problems

- congenital heart problems

- 1/2,000 to 1/30,000 live births

Syndrome Definition . . . .

Pierre Robin sequence is the term given to a birth defect involving micrognathia (underdeveloped lower jaw) and glossoptosis (downward displacement of the tongue). Respiratory obstruction may result and cleft palate is common. Up to 30% of children born with Pierre Robin sequence do not survive due to complications of airway obstruction. Aspiration is the primary cause of death. The prognosis is very good for those babies that survive the first few years of life and do not have multiple malformations.

Pierre Robin is an uncommon condition and prevalence numbers range widely from 1/2,000 to 1/30,000 live births. It was first reported in 1923 and is named for Pierre Robin, a French physician who associated the sequence with breathing problems in affected infants. Pierre Robin varies in severity from patient to patient.

The lower jaw develops rapidly in the 8-10 week period of gestation as does the genioglossus muscle needed to anchor the tongue. The tongue then usually descends from the oropharynx and from between the palatal shelves so that the palate can close fully. In children with Pierre Robin sequence, the jaw is too small to allow the tongue to fall into position, and it can remain displaced in the upper back area of the oropharynx and oral cavity. This may interfere with palatal closure. The resulting cleft palate is characteristically U-shaped at midline, and will affect both the hard and soft palate. Cleft lip is usually not seen in Pierre Robin sequence.

Pierre Robin Sequence is also known as:

- Robin Anomalad
- Cleft Palate, Micrognathia, and Glossoptosis
- Pierre Robin Complex
- Pierre Robin Syndrome

A sequence can be considered Pierre Robin *only* if the causes of the presenting anomalies exist. If there are any other symptoms associated with Pierre Robin sequence, it may then be classified as a *syndrome*. Many genetically-caused syndromes have micrognathia as a characteristic, and this inherited jaw malformation is considered the causation for the Robin sequence. A genetic consultation and team approach to management are both recommended. Robin sequence has been associated specifically with Stickler syndrome, Velocardiofacial syndrome, Treacher Collins syndrome, Trisomy 18, and Fetal Alcohol Syndrome (see *The Source for Syndromes*).

Other physical features of Pierre Robin sequence include congenital heart problems, digital anomalies, defects of the eye, and congenital glaucoma. Ear defects, such as deformities of the pinna, low set ears, external auditory meatus anomalies, and structural defects of the ossicles of the middle ear have also been exhibited. Skeletal defects may also occur.

Behavioral Characteristics Profile . . . .

The behavioral characteristics associated with Pierre Robin sequence are explained in the following section.

Persistent Apnea

Placement of the tongue may obstruct normal breathing in babies with Pierre Robin sequence and may be the cause of apnea. However, sleep apnea has also been reported in wakeful situations. These children should not be placed on their backs to sleep, but should be put in a prone position (on their stomachs) to reduce the possibility of the tongue falling back into the airway.

Central Nervous System Impairment

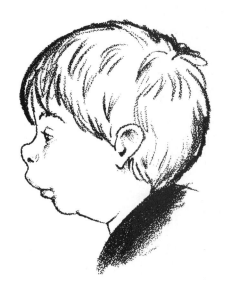

Children with Pierre Robin sequence are at risk for minimal brain dysfunction which often manifests as a learning disability. Cerebral anoxia secondary to upper airway obstruction and hypoxia are the primary causes for damage to the central nervous system.

Mental Retardation

If the hypoxia and upper airway obstruction cause significant brain damage, children may educationally test in the range of mental retard-ation. Hearing impairment may also affect the learning abilities of these children.

Speech-Language Issues . . . .

As an SLP, you should be aware of several specific aspects of the communication profile in Pierre Robin sequence. These aspects are summarized in the following information.

Feeding Difficulties

The structural anomalies resulting from Pierre Robin sequence place an affected child at great risk for feeding difficulties. Because the oral and nasal cavities are part of the respiratory system, and we know that respiratory obstruction may occur, you should be concerned about feeding movements. The possibility of cleft palate will significantly affect feeding. Nasal regurgitation of food/liquids is common. The use of specially-designed cleft palate "squeeze" bottles and other feeding techniques (including positioning) is recommended.

Dysphagia

Dysphagia, or swallowing disorder, may be present in children with Pierre Robin sequence. Up to 30% of children born with Pierre Robin sequence don't survive due to complications of airway obstruction, and aspiration is the primary cause of death. These feeding and swallowing difficulties can result in weight loss and failure to thrive.

Articulation/Voice Disorders

The same structural differences that affect feeding and swallowing movements can affect articulatory movements, speech production, and voice. Any presenting cleft of the hard palate or velum may cause hypernasality and/or nasal emissions. Velopharyngeal insufficiency must be evaluated for causation. Either a cleft problem or palatopharyngeal valving problems or a combination of both should be suspected.

Abnormal compensatory articulation movements may develop as a secondary complication of the palatal and pharyngeal anomalies. Dental abnormalities may also be seen, particularly malocclusions caused by mandibular underdevelopment.

Hearing Loss

Ear defects, such as deformities of the pinna, low-set ears, external auditory meatus anomalies, and structural defects of the middle ear ossicles are observed. Anomalies of the ear and hearing loss are common due to the presenting palatal cleft. Many babies with clefts of the palate are prone to fluid accumulation behind the eardrum. Hearing loss is more common in children with Pierre Robin sequence than in children with an isolated cleft palate.

If middle ear fluid is left untreated, it could lead to a mild, moderate, or severe hearing loss which could be bilateral or unilateral. This is a treatable, conductive loss in most cases. Myringotomy and tympanostomy tubes can be used to treat these clients. Hearing professionals should continually monitor hearing status.

Language Disorders

Delayed onset of language is common in Pierre Robin sequence and can be significant. This delay may (in combination with hearing loss) even be of a fluctuating nature. The language delay may also be attributed to cerebral anoxia secondary to airway obstruction and hypoxia.

Intervention Issues . . . .

Intervention procedures for Pierre Robin sequence will need to be team-based, including professionals from the medical, educational, and therapeutic fields in addition to family members. There may be extensive medical interventions and surgeries within the first few days, months, or years of life. Airway management is the first priority and a tracheostomy may need to be performed as soon as the airway obstruction is identified. Oxygen delivery via a nasopharyngeal cannula may be put into place to increase respiratory function.

Feeding and the structure of the palate may be the next steps for medical treatment and/or surgery. A surgery in which the tongue is sutured to the lower lip can be performed to keep the tongue in a forward and inferior position. Mandibular distraction is a procedure in which the mandible is cut and an external device is put into place, lengthening the jaw bone about 1 to 2 millimeters a day. As the lower jaw is lengthened, new bone forms to fill in the gap. After three to six weeks, the newly-formed bone becomes solid and the device is removed. Due to the rapid growth of the mandible during the first year of life, the profile of some children may look normal by six years of age even without surgeries. The chin angle may still appear to be abnormal.

A gavage or feeding tube may be used to increase nutrition and weight gain in infants with Pierre Robin sequence. Closure of the cleft palate may be delayed until some growth of the oral and nasal cavities has occurred. This allows the opening to be narrower and for more tissue to be utilized to close the cleft. The velum may be closed in a first procedure, and the hard palate may be closed in a later procedure.

Early Intervention

- Perform a team-based early intervention assessment. Due to the frequency of airway obstruction and resulting complications, immediate medical attention is necessary.

- Initiate feeding evaluations and recommendations very early in the infant's life. Introduce positioning, specialized feeding techniques, and recommend surgery to improve the feeding and nutrition intake for each baby.

Hearing Status

- A hearing loss (possibly conductive and fluctuating) is associated with Pierre Robin sequence. Early identification of any loss is important.

- Monitor the hearing mechanism and status of hearing abilities continually due to the otitis media association of clefts. The client may need surgery for the insertion of pressure equalization.

Articulation/Voice Therapy

- Attention to discrimination and production of oral vs. nasal consonants will combine therapies for articulation and resonance.

- Due to decreased mandibular size, articulation practice should focus on fricatives, interdentals, and bilabial phonemes.

- Identify and eliminate hypernasality and nasal emissions to the best of the child's ability based on structural deficits.

Language Therapy

- Use language stimulation for infants, toddlers, and children with Pierre Robin sequence because they are at risk for language delays.

- Encourage caregiver-child interaction strategies with attention to early socio-communicative games.

- If some degree of central nervous system damage or mental retardation is evident, language therapy should be structured to meet individual needs.

Team Approach

- An audiologist is an important team member. Due to the high numbers of children with Pierre Robin sequence who exhibit hearing loss, early evaluation and continual monitoring of hearing status are appropriate.

- As a speech-language pathologist, address voice, articulation, hearing, and language disorders. In addition, you may be responsible for the feeding evaluation and treatment plan, as well as conducting swallowing therapy.

- A neonatologist (a medical doctor who cares for newborns) may be one of the first professionals to see a child affected by Pierre Robin sequence. The child will probably be admitted into the NICU (neonatal intensive care unit) shortly after birth and will become the responsibility of those who daily deal with severely-involved infants.

- The status of the middle ear and any palatal recommendations are the responsibility of an otorhinolarnygologist (ear, nose, and throat doctor). Surgical recommendations may be necessary. Closure of the palate may be needed, but can be delayed until growth of the hard and soft palates occurs.

- Orthodontists can help treat the malocclusion that results from lack of mandibular development.

- A craniofacial team referral can be made upon the birth of a child with Pierre Robin sequence. This team can include many of the professionals mentioned above, but it may only be available in larger metropolitan areas.

Summary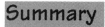

Pierre Robin sequence is a birth defect involving micrognathia (underdeveloped lower jaw) and glossoptosis (downward displacement of the tongue). A resulting cleft palate often occurs due to obstruction of the closing of the palatal shelves in utero. Respiratory obstruction may also result. Up to 30% of children born with Pierre Robin sequence do not survive due to complications of airway obstruction. For those babies who do survive the first few years of life and who do not have multiple malformations, the prognosis is very good.

Associated characteristics of Pierre Robin include possible learning difficulties, ranging from learning disabilities to mental retardation. The cause of these learning difficulties is anoxia secondary to airway obstruction.

Hearing loss is common and is usually treatable. Expect articulation and voice disorders as a result of structural abnormalities. Language development may be delayed with hearing loss and effects of oxygen deprivation considered the primary causes.

A team approach is highly recommended for children with Pierre Robin sequence because so many systems may be affected. Medical, surgical, educational, and therapeutic services are critical, and early intervention is essential.

References . . . .

Batshaw, M. & Perret, Y. *Children with Disabilities—A Medical Primer, Third Edition*. Baltimore, MD: Paul H. Brookes Publishing Co., 1992.

Gerber, S. E. *Etiology and Prevention of Communicative Disorders, Second Edition*. San Diego, CA: Singular Publishing Group, Inc., 1998.

Gilbert, P. *The A-Z Reference Book of Syndromes and Inherited Disorders, Second Edition*. New York, NY: Chapman & Hall, 1996.

"Information about Pierre Robin Sequence." Brochure from the Cleft Palate Foundation, 1990.

Jung, J. *Genetic Syndromes in Communication Disorders*. Austin, TX: Pro-Ed, 1989.

McWilliams, B. J., Moris, H. L., & Shelton, R. L. *Cleft Palate Speech, Second Edition*. Philadelphia, PA: B.C. Decker, Inc., 1990.

"Pierre Robin Sequence Information." <http://www.pierrerobin.org/auses.html> September 18, 1999.

"Pierre Robin Sequence Information." <http://www.neonatology.org/syllabus/pierre.robin.html> April 30, 1999.

Shprintzen, R. J. *Genetics, Syndromes, and Communication Disorders*. San Diego, CA: Singular Publishing Group, Inc., 1997.

Shprintzen, R. J. & Bardach, J. *Cleft Palate Speech Management: A Multidisciplinary Approach*. St. Louis, MO: Mosby Year Book, 1995.

● ● ● ● ● ● ●

Notes . . . .

Stickler Syndrome

Characteristics

- Vision
- Facial features
- Hearing problems
- Bone and joint problems
- Speech and language problems
- Normal life span

Syndrome Definition . . . .

- one of the most common syndromes in the U.S.

- connective tissue disorder

- 1/10,000 live births

- difficult to diagnose

- vision and hearing problems

- bone and joint problems

Stickler syndrome is a fairly common connective tissue disorder caused by a range of collagen gene mutations. It was first studied at the Mayo Clinic by Dr. Stickler in 1965. Characteristics of the syndrome vary widely and to truly diagnose the syndrome, a genetic evaluation is necessary. It's a complicated medical condition due to the variance of symptoms and the high numbers of body systems that can be affected by the syndrome.

Two types of Stickler syndrome have been identified (Hawley, 1999). Type I (also known as Hereditary Progressive Anthroophthalmopathy) is caused by a mutation in a gene on chromosome 12. Type I has vision, joint, craniofacial, and hearing problems. Type II is caused by a mutation on chromosome 6 and does not have the vision problems that Type I does. Stickler syndrome is an autosomal dominant trait, which means that an affected person has a 50% chance of passing it on through birth.

One of the manifestations of a connective tissue disorder is the presence of bone and joint problems. Scoliosis (curvature of the spine), joint pain, arthritis, club foot, vertebral abnormalities, and double jointedness may be present and tend to worsen with age. Problems with the ankles, knees, and wrist bones, and subluxation of the hip may be seen. A cardiac complication (mitral valve prolapse) may also occur.

Stickler Syndrome

Type 1
- also known as Hereditary Progressive Anthroophthalmopathy
- caused by a gene mutation on chromosome 12
- vision, joint, craniofacial, and hearing disorders

Type 2
- caused by a gene mutation on chromosome 6
- same problems as as Type 1, but without the vision disorder

Facial features of Stickler syndrome include mild, midface hypoplasia; a round face; flat cheeks; and maxillary deficiency. An association with Pierre Robin sequence is seen in the presence of cleft palate, micrognathia, and glossoptosis (downward displacement of the tongue). A shorted ramus of the mandible is seen with the micrognathia.

Stickler syndrome is the second most common syndrome associated with cleft palate in absence of cleft lip (Shprintzen, 1997). Anteverted nares, a short nose, and a depressed nasal root may also be exhibited. A congenitally small airway may cause upper airway obstruction and sleep apnea may develop later in life. Vision disorders that can occur with Stickler include nearsightedness, astigmatism, cataracts, retina detachment, and glaucoma. The more serious of these disorders can lead to blindness.

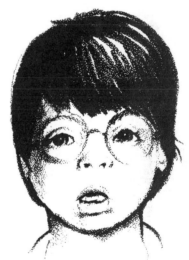

Even though Stickler may be one of the most common syndromes in the United States, it is rarely diagnosed. In other words, many people who have minor symptoms may *never* be identified. Of those who are identified with Stickler, vision and arthritic problems are the most prominent. It's estimated that 1/10,000 people have Stickler syndrome, and that very few of these people know they have it.

A further look at some of the behavioral characteristics associated with Stickler syndrome are explained in this section.

Vision

As mentioned before, people with Type I Stickler exhibit several vision problems including nearsightedness, cataracts, retina detachment, and astigmatism. More serious problems include the deterioration of the gel that fills the eye, eyes moving independently of each other, and glaucoma. Any of these vision problems can lead to blindness.

Facial Features

It's difficult to diagnose Stickler syndrome because many children with the disorder tend have round, cherubic, "cute" faces that often appear normal. In addition, the craniofacial alterations are not particularly stigmatizing. At least one-third of all babies initially diagnosed with Robin sequence have Stickler syndrome (Shprintzen, 2000). Other facial characteristics include mild, midface hypoplasia; flat cheeks; and maxillary deficiency.

Hearing Problems

Hearing loss is a typical symptom of Stickler syndrome. The hearing loss tends to affect either the middle or inner ear. In extreme cases, deafness can result.

Bone and Joint Problems

Stickler syndrome is a connective tissue disorder caused by more than one gene that affects the formation of collagen, a major component of cartilage and connective tissue. Since much of the human body is composed of cartilage and joints, skeletal formation is affected by the syndrome. Problems like scoliosis, arthritis, club foot, and double jointedness may be seen. Pain is frequent in the ankles, wrists, and hips. Many of these symptoms worsen with age.

Speech and Language Problems

Stickler syndrome has major impacts on speech, feeding, hearing, resonance, articulation, and language development. Articulation disorders tend to be secondary to the malocculsion. Tongue-backing, lingual-protrusion, distortions, and micrognathia with or without anterior skeletal open-bites may be seen. More thorough speech-language concerns are discussed in the Speech-Language Issues section.

Normal Life Span

Those with the syndrome are expected to have a normal life span and to perform within normal limits in cognitive and learning tasks. Attention to the vision abilities in early intervention is mandatory for children with Stickler syndrome to achieve their full potential. Prognosis depends on the timing of treatment and the severity of the associated disabilities.

Speech-Language Issues . . . .

There are many speech and language issues to be aware of when working with someone with Stickler syndrome.

Hearing Impairment

The syndrome is strongly associated with hearing impairments. The external ear may be low-set, with 10-12% of cases having auricular malformations (Jung, 1989). Middle ear anomalies are rare, unless they exist secondary to cleft palate. Chronic, serious otitis media has been reported. A bilateral conductive loss in a mild to severe range may be seen. A high-frequency sensorineural loss is found in 15-20% of sufferers (Shprintzen, 1997). Deafness can result in extreme cases.

Hearing complications can lead to difficulties in several language areas including receptive skills, developing a lexicon, marking morphemes, and pragmatics. The length and complexity of expressive language may also be affected by hearing difficulties.

Early Feeding Complications

Palatal and pharyngeal structure anomalies and velopharyngeal insufficiencies present difficulties for infants with Stickler syndrome in the area of feeding. Sucking and swallowing can also be affected. Because sucking and swallowing are prespeech movements, they should be evaluated as soon as complications are suspected.

Resonance Disorders

Hypernasality is the most common resonance disorder due to the high percentage of people with Stickler syndrome who also have a cleft palate or velopharyngeal insufficiency. Submucous clefting is also seen and may be more difficult to diagnose than the cleft of the hard or soft palate. Cleft lip is not common. Hyponasality, or denasality, may be exhibited in patients due to a small nasal capsule and a small nasopharyngeal area.

Articulation Errors

Articulation errors are secondary to the malocclusion caused by maxillary dysplasia and/or micrognathia. Lip closure may make it difficult to produce bilabial consonants. Oral and nasal contrast in articulatory production may not be developed. Substitutions at the level of the glottis or within the pharynx may occur for oral anterior sounds, and nasal continuants may be substituted for oral continuants. These could be considered compensatory articulation errors secondary to cleft palate and velopharyngeal insufficiency.

Language Development

Language develops within normal limits for the majority of those with Stickler syndrome. Introduce appropriate language stimulation strategies as needed.

Intervention Issues . . . .

Because Stickler is so difficult to diagnose, and because such a large percentage of those affected by the syndrome are never diagnosed, don't depend on a first diagnosis to chart your intervention. Rather, look at various symptoms according to *obvious disabilities*. Medical intervention with emphasis on a team approach is required because Stickler is such a complicated syndrome.

Early Intervention

- Early intervention with infants, toddlers, and preschoolers should include a team approach that involves the child's family.

- Feeding evaluation and management may be one of the earliest interventions to consider with Stickler syndrome due to the craniofacial differences.

- Eye examinations should be conducted as early as possible due to the high percentage of vision impairments.

Hearing Status

- An audiologist should conduct early identification of any hearing impairment to determine the level and type of hearing loss.

- Continually monitor hearing status, particularly the middle ear status for episodes of otitis media.

- Surgery for auricular deformations may be needed.

- Medical intervention may have to be performed and amplification may need to be provided.

Palatal Competency

- Identify cleft palate, submucous cleft, or velopharyngeal insufficiency as early as possible. Any structural anomalies will affect feeding, pre-speech movements, and airway competence.

- Surgeries may be necessary prior to beginning articulation or voice therapy.

Articulation/Voice Therapy

- A therapy focus on discrimination and production of oral and nasal consonants will address both the articulation and resonance areas.

- Target production of consonants affected by malocclusion, particularly fricatives.

- Monitor phonemes affected by any hearing impairment.

- Address the client's rate of speech, if necessary.

Language Stimulation

- Language stimulation may be necessary in both the receptive and expressive areas, depending on the degree of hearing impairment.

- Give special attention to written language and compensatory strategies due to the wide range of possible vision difficulties found in Stickler syndrome.

Team Approach

- Have ophthalmologic professionals consult for the assessment and treatment of vision difficulties.

- Orthopedic consultation can address the bone and joint problems.

- As the SLP, you are needed for feeding evaluations, resonance assessment, and treatment of voice and articulation disorders.

- Audiologists can assess and perform management duties for suspected hearing impairment.

Genetic Counseling

- Since Stickler syndrome is an autosomal dominant trait and can be passed on through birth, genetic counseling is recommended.

Summary ·

Stickler syndrome is a connective tissue disorder caused by a range of collagen gene mutations. Two types of Stickler have been identified, and each has a distinct etiology in chromosome mutation. The syndrome is grossly underdiagnosed, and many affected persons may never know they have the syndrome.

Primary characteristics of the syndrome include visual disorders, orthopedic disorders, and specific craniofacial features. These disorders can range from mild to severe.

A team approach to intervention is recommended, especially medical personnel, because Stickler is a complicated medical condition. Speech-language pathologists are primary members of the team due to feeding, speech, and voice issues. Because there are associated hearing impairments, audiologists will also participate on the team.

References . . . .

Batshaw, M. & Perret, Y. *Children with Disabilities—A Medical Primer, Third Edition.* Baltimore, MD: Paul H. Brookes Publishing Co., 1992.

Gerber, S. E. *Etiology and Prevention of Communicative Disorders, Second Edition.* San Diego, CA: Singular Publishing Group, Inc., 1998.

Gilbert, P. *The A-Z Reference Book of Syndromes and Inherited Disorders, Second Edition.* New York, NY: Chapman & Hall, 1996.

Hawley, D. "Stickler Syndrome Page." <http://member.aol.com/dhawley/stickler.html> July 21, 1999.

Jung, J. *Genetic Syndromes in Communication Disorders.* Austin, TX: Pro-Ed, 1989.

McWilliams, B. J., Moris, H. L., & Shelton, R. L. *Cleft Palate Speech, Second Edition.* Philadelphia, PA: B.C. Decker, Inc., 1990.

Pore, S. G. & Reed, K. L. *Quick Reference to Speech-Language Pathology.* Gaithersburg, MD: Aspen Publishers, Inc., 1999.

Shprintzen, R. J. *Syndrome Identification for Speech-Language Pathology.* San Diego, CA: Singular Publishing Group, Inc., 2000.

Shprintzen, R. J. *Genetics, Syndromes, and Communication Disorders.* San Diego, CA: Singular Publishing Group, Inc., 1997.

Shprintzen, R. J. & Bardach, J. *Cleft Palate Speech Management: A Multidisciplinary Approach.* St. Louis, MO: Mosby Year Book, 1995.

●　　　●　　　●　　　●　　　●　　　●　　　●

Notes . . . .

Sturge-Weber Syndrome

Characteristics

- Seizures
- Hemiplegia
- Vision impairment
- Malocclusion
- Mental retardation

- port wine birthmark on one side of the face

- both genders affected equally

- overgrowth of tissues and skeleton

- seizures and convulsions

- articulation problems

- mental retardation

- glaucoma

Syndrome Definition . . . .

Sturge-Weber syndrome is classified as a neurocutaneous syndrome, which means there is a combination of skin abnormalities, seizures, and cognitive deficits associated with the disorder (Batshaw & Perret, 1992). Etiology is unknown, but it is considered a non-inherited, sporadic mutation. Exact incidence figures are also unknown, but the syndrome is considered rare. Both genders are affected equally.

The most noticeable characteristic at birth is a port wine birthmark on one side of the baby's face that touches at least one upper eyelid and the forehead. Color of the birthmark can vary from pink to deep purple based on the number of abnormal blood vessels under the surface of the skin. The port wine birthmark often indicates neurological problems because the blood vessel malformation on the skin is also present in the brain, leading to cortical atrophy on that side. Intracranial calcifications will be visible on X-ray scans in the temporal and occipital areas of the affected side of the brain when the child is over two years old.

Hyperplasia, or an overgrowth of the maxillary process, is unusual, but does occur. The increased blood flow to the craniofacial area causes an overgrowth of all tissues, including the skeleton. The hyperplasia primarily affects the maxillary process but can extend into the jaw and tongue as well.

This results in a malocclusion (bad closure) of the jaw, which causes articulation problems (Shprintzen, 1997).

Congenital glaucoma occurs in about 30% of Sturge-Weber cases (Le Postollec, 1998), but is usually restricted to only the eye affected by the port wine stain. The hypervascularization of the craniofacial complex can lead to increased pressure in the eye involved with the blood flow anomalies.

Seizures with convulsions are also part of the syndrome. The seizures often begin when the child is around one year old. They occur on the *opposite* side

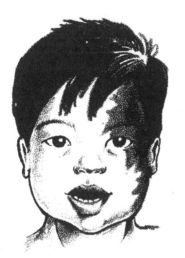

of the body from the birthmark. Neurological findings can also indicate paralysis or paresis on the side of the body which has the seizures. The weakening or loss of body use on that side coincides with the convulsions, which can vary in severity. The seizures are often difficult to control with antiepileptic drugs. The more severe convulsive seizure cases may result in the need for a hemispherectomy (removal of the damaged half of the brain). This surgical procedure removes the aberrant portion of the brain which is disrupting function, allowing the other hemisphere to develop dominance.

Most children with the syndrome have mental retardation. The cognitive impairment can cause developmental problems in acquisition of speech-language skills, motor abilities, and pre-academic readiness for learning. The complicating factor of seizures can further affect the developmental process or compromise acquired skills.

Behavioral Characteristics Profile . . . .

Here are the behavioral characteristics associated with Sturge-Weber syndrome.

Seizures

The seizure component usually begins around one year of age. The severity of the seizures varies, and the convulsive aspect can be frightening. The neurological implications of the seizures can be extremely debilitating—erasing developmental progress in some areas and minimizing further acquisition of skills. If medication is not effective in controlling seizures, more extreme surgical intervention may be necessary. This only adds more complications to the progressive developmental problems.

Hemiplegia

Children with Sturge-Weber usually experience a weakness or paralysis on one side of the body—the side opposite the port wine birthmark. Humans are neurologically wired for a cross-lateral dominance, so the brain hemisphere affected by the vascular abnormalities controls movement in the opposite side of the body. The hemiplegia contributes to developmental delays in acquisition of motor skills in both fine and gross motor areas. Developmental milestones are often delayed and compromised by the neurological involvement.

Vision Impairment

The abnormal vascular supply indicated by the port wine birthmark usually affects the eye on the side of the birthmark. The child's eyes can be different colors because of the aberrant blood vessel present at the back of the eye. Glaucoma (measured by high pressure in the eye) usually occurs at birth but can develop during the preschool years. Glaucoma will be present in the eye on the same side as the birthmark and can lead to blindness if left untreated.

Malocclusion

The abnormal jaw alignment can result in both resonance and sound production errors. The size and shape parameters of the oral cavity may not be balanced symmetrically on both sides. This is challenging to a child trying to balance resonance and trying to produce various phonemes.

Mental Retardation

Developmental abnormalities are evidenced consistent with the degree of mental retardation. Developmental milestones will be affected by both the neurological complications and cognitive impairment.

Speech-Language Issues

• Articulation

• Voice

• Language

Speech-Language Issues . . . .

Speech-language issues in Sturge-Weber syndrome are secondary to the unilateral maxillary hyperplasia and degree of cognitive impairment. These two variables can significantly affect the development of vocal quality, articulation, and language abilities. Hearing acuity is usually normal.

Articulation

The acquisition of correct sound production patterns can be affected by the neurological weakness or paralysis, as well as structural deviations that can occur on the side of the mouth which has the port wine birthmark. The malocclusion can lead to inaccurate mouth postures or compensatory movements which compromise intelligibility. Muscle weakness on one side of the mouth can further challenge oral-motor production of sounds.

Voice

The syndrome can affect secondary aspects of vocal production. Hoarseness can result from excessive tension to compensate for hemiplegia in vocal cord function. Hyponasality has been noted in some children secondary to nasal obstruction caused by the excessive tissue growth associated with the hypervascularization (Shprintzen, 1997). Balance of nasal resonance in vocal quality can also be deviant if significant variations exist in the maxillary structures for one side of the face.

Language

Language delays are consistent with the extent of mental retardation. It is usual to experience developmental delays across all areas of language acquisition during the developmental years. Stimulation will be necessary in both receptive and expressive communication skills to accomplish a language developmental age commensurate with a child's mental age level.

Intervention for Sturge-Weber syndrome will focus on secondary deficits. Delays in all areas of development are likely due to the neurological involvement and ongoing nature of aspects of the syndrome such as seizures, glaucoma, hemiplegia, and mental retardation. However, early intervention can dramatically improve a child's acquisition of basic language and motor skills when initiated as soon as possible following diagnosis.

Articulation

- Teach articulation of specific sounds using an oral-motor approach for positioning the articulators.

- Teach compensatory movements and postures to improve intelligibility.

- Teach oral exercises to strengthen musculature if weakness or paralysis is present on half of the body.

- Prosthetic and orthodontic intervention may need to accompany articulation intervention.

Voice

- Emphasize breath support and easy onset of phonation to prevent excessive tension. This will accomplish volume and vocal fold closure when speaking.

- Introduce good general vocal hygiene habits to parents, teachers, and the child to prevent abusive vocal habits from developing.

- Reinforce resonance balance with palatal exercises to strengthen velopharyngeal closure.

- Goals should be consistent with organic capabilities and take into account structural and neurological limitations. Surgical intervention may be necessary if tissue obstructions are present.

Intervention Issues

- Articulation

- Voice

- Language

- Vision

- Team Approach

Language

- Stimulate receptive and expressive language as early as possible. Developmental delays may be overcome with early intervention and focused introduction of foundation language skills.

- Present language using multi-sensory techniques and using suggestions from occupational and physical therapy to stimulate the neurology and circumvent muscle weaknesses. Involve the whole body in the learning process and introduce materials in natural contexts.

- Mediate language level by the level of cognitive functioning. The degree of mental retardation will impact goals and functional levels.

Vision

- Visual deficits may not be significant, but compensatory teaching should include other sensory channels when possible to make up for any visual problems.

- Present materials to favor the unaffected eye, if necessary.

Team Approach

- An ophthamologist will monitor and control glaucoma with eyedrops or surgery. Without treatment, progressive deterioration of vision in the affected eye can lead to blindness.

- A physician or neurologist will be critical in controlling seizures and preventing further brain damage or loss of acquired skills. If anti-convulsant drugs are ineffective, surgery may be necessary on the affected area of the brain.

- Physical and occupational therapy can help compensate for motor developmental deficits secondary to hemiplegia. Goals should work to develop general strength, range of motion, and applied functional skills through motor patterning.

- Psychological counseling may be necessary to assist a child in coping with the facial disfiguration of the birthmark. As a child grows older, the self-consciousness regarding appearance can lead to withdrawal and social problems.

Summary ·

Sturge-Weber syndrome is noticeable at birth by the port wine birthmark on the infant's face. It's not always diagnosed until the seizure aspect of the disorder is evidenced during the first or second year. Initial neurological and x-ray scans may be negative for components. The associated abnormalities are often detected only after the brain begins growing.

If only the skin of the face is involved, the impact of Sturge-Weber is fairly limited with little threat to general health. However, if the disease is more extensive and affects blood vessels in the brain, seizures can be a serious complication with life-threatening implications. In addition to seizures, the abnormal blood supply (causing the discoloration of the skin) can cause glaucoma, hemiplegia, abnormal tissue growth of the maxillary process, and mental retardation.

The primary medical components of the syndrome trigger general developmental delays that can be progressive without effective medical and educational intervention. Secondary problems include deficits in articulation, vocal production and quality, language development, vision, gross and fine motor skills, learning, and emotional well-being. Complete recovery in cases of Sturge-Weber syndrome is unlikely, but improved treatment techniques and cosmetic surgery make the future much brighter.

● ● ● ● ● ● ●

References

Batshaw, M. & Perret, Y. *Children with Disabilities—A Medical Primer, Third Edition.* Baltimore, MD: Paul H. Brookes Publishing Co., 1992.

Gilbert, P. *The A-Z Reference Book of Syndromes and Inherited Disorders, Second Edition.* New York, NY: Chapman & Hall, 1996.

Le Postollec, M. "Byron's Battle with Sturge-Weber Syndrome." *ADVANCE for Speech-Language Pathologists & Audiologists*, April 20, 1998.

Shprintzen, R. J. *Genetics, Syndromes, and Communication Disorders.* San Diego, CA: Singular Publishing Group, Inc., 1997.

Sturge-Weber Foundation: 1-800-627-5482.

Treacher Collins Syndrome

Characteristics

- Hearing loss
- Normal cognition
- Normal life expectancy

- autosomal dominant inheritance

- both genders affected equally

- anomalies present at birth

- severe craniofacial anomalies

- possible heart defects

- downslanting eyes

Syndrome Definition . . . .

Treacher Collins syndrome is a relatively rare genetic disorder that follows an autosomal dominant pattern of inheritance. This means that the gene may be inherited or may be the result of a mutation. A single gene on the long arm of chromosome 5 is the chromosomal site. Those who carry the gene have a 50/50 chance of bearing a child with Treacher Collins.

The first case of the syndrome was described in 1846. In 1900, a British ophthalmologist named Dr. Treacher Collins gave a definitive diagnosis, and thus the syndrome was named. It affects males and females equally, and the associated anomalies are present at birth.

Characteristics of the syndrome include mild to severe craniofacial signs. Underdevelopment of the facial skeleton is the most prominent feature. Hearing loss is highly evident with malformations of the outer and middle ear occurring frequently. Possible heart defects have also been noted. Early differentiation between Treacher Collins syndrome and Goldenhar syndrome can be difficult because they present the same phenotype.

Characteristic facial appearance includes mandibular and maxillary hypoplasia including the zygomatic arches, downslanting eyes (palpebral fissures), a long face, and a beak-like nose. Cleft palate and/or cleft lip, an anterior skeletal open bite, and hypoplasia of the teeth may also occur. A small, narrow pharyngeal area results in airway obstruction and apnea, as well as feeding and eating problems. An unusual hairline of a long extension of hair onto the cheek area is common.

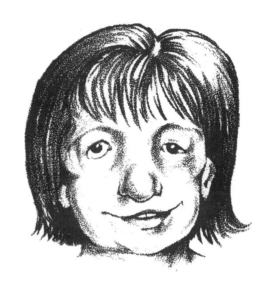

In addition to the downslanting eyes and coloboma (clefts) of the lower eyelid, total or partial absence of lower eyelashes may be evident, as well as strabismus and astigmatism of the eye.

Behavioral Characteristics Profile . . . .

The behavioral characteristics associated with Treacher Collins syndrome are explained in the following section.

> **Treacher Collins Syndrome** is also known as:
>
> - Mandibulofacial Dysostosis
>
> - Franceschetti-Zwahlen-Klein Syndrome
>
> - Treacher Collins-Franceshetti Syndrome

Hearing Loss

The hearing loss most frequently associated with Treacher Collins syndrome is bilateral and conductive. Occasional sensorineural losses are reported. Early identification of hearing loss is highly recommended.

Speech-Language Issues

- Hearing Impairment

- Voice Disorders

- Articulation Disorders

- Feeding Disorders/ Dysphagia

- Hearing Loss

Cognition within Normal Limits

Approximately 5% of the population with Treacher Collins have been diagnosed with some type of mental retardation. Otherwise, cognitive development parallels that of the non-affected population.

Normal Life Expectancy

Abnormal neck posturing and altered sleep patterns including sleep apnea frequently occur in those with Treacher Collins syndrome. Tracheostomy is sometimes needed in extreme cases of airway obstruction. Life span is expected within normal limits when the upper airway obstruction is resolved.

Speech-Language Issues . . . .

Children identified at birth with Treacher Collins syndrome are immediately at risk for speech-language disorders due to craniofacial and hearing structural anomalies.

Hearing Impairment

Bilateral, conductive hearing loss is reported in almost all affected by Treacher Collins syndrome, with 85% having pinna malformations (Jung, 1989). These can range from minor malformations (including helical thinning) to complete microtia. There may be external auditory canal atresia (underdevelopment and closure), preauricular ear tags, and the absence of external meatus (Jung, 1989). Ossicular anomalies are common, including fixation of the footplate of the stapes. Occasional sensorineural loss may occur.

Voice Disorders

Voice disorders are usually in the nasal resonance area. Muffled resonance and hyponasality are due to a small nasopharynx and choanal atresia or stenosis. Mixed resonance with hyponasality and hypernasality with nasal air emission can occur due to velopharyngeal insufficiency combined with nasal obstructions.

Articulation Disorders

Several specific articulation disorders have been associated with Treacher Collins syndrome, and they are secondary to the structural anomalies of the facial skeleton and the upper airway. Severe tongue backing may be produced due to severe micrognathia. The anterior skeletal open bite will affect articulation, particularly the production of bilabials, fricatives, and affricates. Substitution of glottal stops for stop/plosives occurs and other articulation errors may be attempts to compensate for voice disorders.

Feeding Disorders/Dysphagia

Feeding and swallowing difficulties are common in children with Treacher Collins syndrome. Sucking, swallowing, nasal regurgitation of food, and mastication abilities may all be affected by the structural anomalies.

Hearing Loss

Language development is at risk for children with Treacher Collins syndrome secondary to the presenting hearing loss. The development and use of the syntactic morphemes and age-appropriate semantics is important for the child with a prelinguistic loss.

Intervention for Treacher Collins revolves around surgical management of craniofacial anomalies and associated difficulties. A team approach is critical, with significant roles for the speech-language pathologist and audiologist.

Intervention Issues

- Hearing Impairments

- Craniofacial Malformations

- Articulation Therapy

- Voice Therapy

- Language Stimulation

- Genetic Counseling

- Team Approach

Hearing Impairments

- An audiologist should identify any hearing loss as soon as possible and should provide appropriate amplification early in the child's life.

- Note that surgeries may be necessary to reconstruct the outer ear, the auditory canal, and/or the middle ear.

- Monitor ongoing hearing status.

- Include aural rehabilitation or habilitation training in your treatment plan.

Craniofacial Malformations

- Note that early reconstructive surgery may be needed to redirect facial skeletal growth. Surgical alteration of the maxilla or mandible can normalize the jaw relationship and improve the oral cavity for speech production, particularly for fricatives, affricates, bilabials, labiodentals, and lingua-alveolars.

- Note that surgery to relieve upper airway obstruction will affect both oral and nasal resonance.

- Be aware that pharyngeal flap surgery may be contraindicated in Treacher Collins syndrome due to the fact that the flap may compromise the airway.

- Use a prosthetic device to reduce the hypernasal voice production, although there may be limits as to the final result.

Articulation Therapy

- Use traditional articulation therapy and behavioral modification programs to improve articulatory competence.

- Take structural differences into consideration in therapeutic management.

- Include bilabials, fricatives, affricates, and labiodentals as speech targets.

Voice Therapy

- Reduction of abnormal voice production in both oral and nasal resonance will depend on the presenting structure. Target maximum oral production and reduce nasality depending on the degree of velopharyngeal closure.

- Note that the client may have to have a tonsillectomy to reduce hyponasality.

Language Stimulation

- Early intervention, early identification, and early management of hearing abilities and language stimulation are recommended for all children with Treacher Collins syndrome.

- Monitor parent-infant interaction and attachment to make sure communication development is ongoing.

- Emphasize use of morphemes in treatment and stress their ongoing development.

- Develop a lexicon rich in substantive and relational words.

Genetic Counseling

- Because someone affected with Treacher Collins has a 50% chance of producing an affected child, genetic counseling may be needed.

Team Approach

- Use a variety of professionals to work with the family and affected child. Early intervention and early care are highly recommended.

- Craniofacial team services can provide a needed continuum of services.

Summary · · · · · · · · · · · · · · · · · ·

Treacher Collins syndrome is a genetic disorder characterized by an autosomal dominant transmission pattern of inheritance. The major characteristics of the syndrome are mild to severe craniofacial anomalies. The underdevelopment of the maxilla, mandible, cheekbone, and unusual eye structure are easily identifiable as Treacher Collins syndrome. Ear malformations are common and of a wide variety.

Children with Treacher Collins syndrome are at-risk for speech-language development, especially articulation and voice. Multiple misarticulations and vocal quality disorders are also seen. Bilateral (mild, conductive) hearing loss is most common. Language disorders may also occur as a result of the hearing impairment.

Children affected by Treacher Collins syndrome are best served through a team approach, with a craniofacial team making recommendations for surgeries and treatments. Speech-language pathologists and audiologists will be primary team members in interventions.

References . . . .

Batshaw, M. & Perret, Y. *Children with Disabilities—A Medical Primer, Third Edition.* Baltimore, MD: Paul H. Brookes Publishing Co., 1992.

Carlucci, D. *Minor Considerations: Diagnosing Minor Craniofacial Anomalies.* ADVANCE for Speech-Language Pathologists & Audiologists, 1999.

Gerber, S. E. *Etiology and Prevention of Communicative Disorders, Second Edition.* San Diego, CA: Singular Publishing Group, Inc., 1998.

Gilbert, P. *The A-Z Reference Book of Syndromes and Inherited Disorders, Second Edition.* New York, NY: Chapman & Hall, 1996.

Jung, J. H. *Genetic Syndromes in Communication Disorders.* Austin, TX: Pro-Ed., 1989.

McWilliams, B. J., Moris, H. L., & Shelton, R. L. *Cleft Palate Speech, Second Edition.* Philadelphia, PA: B.C. Decker, Inc., 1990.

Pore, S. G. & Reed, K. L. *Quick Reference to Speech-Language Pathology.* Gaithersburg, MD: Aspen Publishers, Inc., 1999.

Shprintzen, R. J. *Genetics, Syndromes, and Communication Disorders.* San Diego, CA: Singular Publishing Group, Inc., 1997.

Shprintzen, R. J. & Bardach, J. *Cleft Palate Speech Management: A Multidisciplinary Approach.* St. Louis, MO: Mosby, 1995.

"The Treacher Collins Network." <http://www.geocities.com/Heartland/Plains/6153/> August 31, 1999.

Usher Syndrome

Characteristics

- Hearing impairments
- Vision impairments
- Ataxia
- Mental retardation
- Emotional episodes

- deafness or significant hearing loss

- gradual loss of vision

- 3-5/100,000 births

- males and females affected equally

- mental retardation

Syndrome Definition . . . .

Usher syndrome is an inherited syndrome typically linked to congenital deafness/profound hearing loss and severe vision impairments. The disorder has a genetic autosomal recessive cause with a 25% chance of recurrence in siblings. The two primary diagnostic features are severe sensorineural hearing loss or deafness at birth and retinitis pigmentosa (progressive loss of vision caused by abnormal pigment in the cells of the retina).

Incidence ranges from 3-5 per 100,000 births. Males and females appear to be affected equally. It does not appear to be common among African Americans, Asians, or Native Americans. Life span is normal. Some children will also have mental retardation.

Usher syndrome accounts for about 10% of the children who are born deaf, and it is a primary diagnosis for many deaf and blind people. The hearing loss is usually the first symptom to onset, with retinitis pigmentosa occurring in the second decade of life. (An interesting counterpart to Usher is Refsum syndrome, which also has both hearing and vision loss, but with an opposite onset pattern i.e., retinitis pigmentosa usually occurs first and hearing loss begins in the second or third decade of life, progressing to a severe-profound level.)

Types of Usher Syndrome

Type 1
- absence of vestibular function
- abnormal motor developmental milestones, evidenced by delays in sitting and walking

Type 2
- mild hearing loss in low frequencies
- profound hearing loss or deafness in higher frequencies

Type 3
- those of Finnish descent display progressive hearing loss at 5 to 10 years of age

There are at least three types of Usher syndrome and they are determined by the severity of the hearing loss and visual impairment. Children who have Type I Usher suffer an absence of vestibular function. This group also demonstrates abnormal motor developmental milestones, evidenced by delays in sitting and walking.

Children who have Type II Usher have a milder audiological impact with a sloping audiogram showing mild hearing loss in low frequencies and profound hearing loss or deafness in higher frequencies. Type III Usher occurs primarily in those of Finnish descent, and they sometimes display progressive hearing loss with onset between 5 to 10 years of age. Type III is similar to Acadian Usher syndrome.

Behavioral Characteristics Profile . . . .

The behavioral characteristics associated with Usher syndrome are explained in the following section.

Hearing Impairments

Congenital sensorineural hearing impairment is one of the hallmark features (90% of Usher syndrome). Hearing loss is typically characterized as severe-profound or deaf, but some types of Usher vary in the actual configuration of impairment. Type II children demonstrate severe-profound loss in higher frequencies, but suffer less severity in lower frequencies. Hearing loss is usually profound, but not progressive.

Vision Impairments

Retinitis pigmentosa is progressive and may eventually result in complete blindness. Night blindness is often the first sign of a visual deterioration that leads to complete loss of vision in about half of those with Usher. Vision problems can onset early but usually are not noticeable until the teenage and young-adult years. In other words, vision is normal at birth but it gradually becomes more difficult to see in the dark and/or have peripheral vision. Cataracts and glaucoma (high pressure within the eyeball) can also occur.

Ataxia

It's important to check certain motor movements in a child to assess for poor balance because ataxia is a possible deficit. For example, have the child turn his head quickly, stand on one foot, or perform other balance tasks. Delays in developmental milestones for sitting, standing, walking, etc. can be another indicator of ataxia in young children. Any child with a significant congenital hearing impairment should be evaluated for balance functions to check for the syndrome.

Mental Retardation

Developmental abnormalities should be monitored closely during the preschool years. Most abnormalities will be associated with poor balance (ataxia) and the significant hearing impairment, but general global delays could indicate mental retardation. The significant sensory issues of Usher syndrome are then further compounded by cognitive limitations. Compensatory strategies should be explored to accomplish academic learning.

Emotional Episodes

Literature on Usher sometimes mentions a co-occurrence of psychosis or mental illness with the disorder but there is not agreement among experts as to whether this is true. Some professionals feel that the psychotic

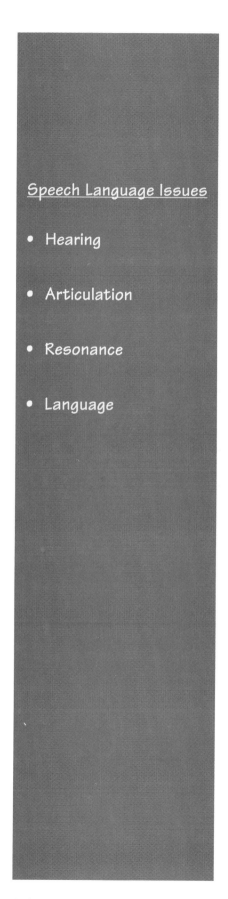

episodes are misrepresented, and are actually emotional reactions to losing two primary sensory systems at a young age. Gilbert (1996) mentioned Hallgren's syndrome as a similar disorder that includes signs of mental instability but is sometimes misdiagnosed as Usher syndrome. It's important to help the child maintain a positive outlook to prevent depression and other psychological responses to the degenerative aspects of the disorder.

Speech-Language Issues . . . .

Speech-language issues in Usher syndrome are caused by the severe sensorineural hearing impairment at birth. Newborn/infant screening programs can have a critical impact on the diagnosis. The sooner the hearing loss is detected and diagnosed, the better the long-term prognosis. Professionals can begin focusing intervention efforts on the aspects of speech-language development that are likely to be affected by the profound hearing impairment.

Hearing

The severity of the sensorineural hearing loss can vary depending on the actual subtype of the syndrome, but it is usually severe and present at birth. The degree of loss can range from moderate to complete deafness, with the possibility of a sloping audiogram which documents the most severe impairment in the high frequency levels. Audiologic evaluations should consistently monitor hearing levels, and compensatory strategies should be implemented as soon as possible to circumvent the hearing deficit.

Articulation

Production of sounds for expressive communication will be significantly impacted by the loss of hearing. Hearing aids might compensate to allow an auditory model for some sounds, but in most children, intelligibility is extremely poor. Alternative augmentative methods for expressive communication are necessary. It's also important to insure that the alternative choice of communication is *not* overly dependent on visual skills, since eventual loss of vision is probable.

Resonance

Voice production is usually within normal parameters in Usher syndrome, but resonance balance can be severely impaired by the hearing loss. Vocal quality is typical of children with deafness or severe-profound hearing loss.

Language

Language development will be affected by the hearing loss. Use compensatory techniques to establish an alternative augmentative system that allows comprehension and expression of basic vocabulary terms, concepts, and needs. Academic learning can be significantly impacted if a solid language foundation is not stabilized during the preschool years. Sign language, picture communication, and other visualization strategies can be used early, but gradual transition to tactile input should be realized in anticipation of reduced visual acuity over time.

Intervention Issues . . . .

Intervention for Usher syndrome revolves primarily around hearing and vision deficits. Compensatory techniques will be important to promote normal development and learning. Establishing a communication system can be very challenging due to the combined vision and hearing impairments. Remediation should be global to encourage as much independence as possible. The child will need to learn how to adapt to the environment and function as productively as possible.

Hearing

- If the child is a candidate for amplification, select an appropriate hearing aid for this type of sensorineural loss.

- Consider amplification for environmental sound awareness to address safety concerns. Some people with Usher have undergone cochlear implants, but more research is needed to thoroughly evaluate whether or not children with the disorder are good candidates for this procedure. However, with the impending loss of vision, hearing enhancement is important.

Augmentative and Alternative Communication

- Explore sign language or a total communication approach that includes as many sensory channels as possible.

- Use visual communication systems initially, but gradually use tactile methods because of the eventual reduction in vision. Visual stimulation may facilitate development of simple sound/word production early in intervention but it should be faded as a primary input system for comprehension. Input should be multi-modal with emphasis on tactile to circumvent the hearing and vision disorders.

Vision

- Fade emphasis on visual input for learning due to the degeneration of vision.

- Initiate compensatory techniques in therapy for the gradual loss of vision within various settings (e.g., school, home, and community).

Language

- Receptive and expressive language acquisition will be critical to development. Introduce and emphasize functional language through sensory exploration. The foundation of language should begin immediately due to the hearing deficits. Language forms the foundation for academic learning, and prognosis will be significantly impacted by whether comprehension and expressive language can be established.

- Language techniques should be consistent with principles of deaf education (i.e., use multisensory stimulation at an early age to develop awareness of semantic meanings through concrete experiences).

- Language levels should be mediated at the cognitive level. If mental retardation is present, communication acquisition will be compromised further than the deficit levels precipitated by hearing and visual problems.

Team Approach

- Audiologists should conduct periodic evaluations to monitor the child's hearing loss, particularly if it becomes worse. They should also assess possible benefits like amplification or cochlear implants.

- An ophthamologist will need to conduct periodic vision evaluations. Retinitis pigmentosa is not always evident at birth and not usually detected in its early stages without very specific examination of the eyes. An ophthamologist should monitor the degenerative aspect of vision to help the child, parents, and educators adjust.

- A teacher trained in deaf education should be the primary classroom consideration or should consult heavily on educational techniques to ensure learning.

- Involve a teacher of the visually impaired based on the degree of deficits evidenced at various stages in the educational process. Introduce compensatory techniques early while residual vision can still help the child learn the modifications.

- Psychological counseling may be necessary for both the parents and child. It's important to explain the degenerative process so the child can prepare for the profound changes that will occur through life. Concern for the physical safety and psychological well-being of the child should be a focus.

Summary . . . .

Usher syndrome is a genetic disorder characterized by significant hearing and visual impairments. The sensorineural hearing loss occurs at birth in 90% of the cases and ranges from moderate to complete deafness. Visual impairment tends to begin in childhood and gradually worsens, regressing to blindness for many. A child with Usher syndrome can be severely disabled in both vision and hearing by young adulthood.

Early specialized teaching can circumvent later problems. It's important to evaluate infants who are deaf or who have severely profound hearing impairments at birth for Usher syndrome so preventative measures can be taken to compensate for hearing and vision difficulties. Intervention efforts should focus on making sure functional skills allow the individual to remain as self-sufficient as possible in later years.

Use communication and teaching methods that maximize multisensory input in early intervention efforts and gradually work toward tactile input as the long-term modality. The immediate concern at the preschool level is to build a solid language foundation despite the significant hearing impairment. Work in conjunction with audiologists and other professionals to insure maximum stimulation before visual deficits compromise learning channels.

Further complications can include mental retardation, ataxia (poor balance), and additional visual complications (e.g., glaucoma, cataracts). Emotional difficulties are not unusual as a child attempts to cope with the regressive nature of the disorder and the frustration of losing two main sensory systems early in life. It's important to be honest and not withhold information from the child. Emphasize the positive aspects of compensatory skills learned. An early diagnosis enhances the opportunities for professionals to assist the child in preparing to cope with Usher syndrome complications later in life.

●　　　●　　　●　　　●　　　●　　　●　　　●

References

Batshaw, M. & Perret, Y. *Children with Disabilities—A Medical Primer, Third Edition*. Baltimore, MD: Paul H. Brookes Publishing Co., 1992.

Gilbert, P. *The A-Z Reference Book of Syndromes and Inherited Disorders, Second Edition*. New York, NY: Chapman & Hall, 1996.

Samuelson, S. & Zahn, J. "Usher's Syndrome." *Ophthalmic Pediatrics and Genetics*, Vol. 2, pp. 71-76, 1990.

Scott, A. "Usher Syndrome." *ADVANCE for Speech-Language Pathologists & Audiologists*, February 16, 1998.

Shprintzen, R. J. *Genetics, Syndromes, and Communication Disorders*. San Diego, CA: Singular Publishing Group, Inc., 1997.

Notes . . . .

Velocardiofacial Syndrome

Characteristics

- Infant feeding problems
- Learning disabilities
- Mental retardation
- Mental illness

- 1/700 live births

- most common cleft palate syndrome

- heart defects

- learning disabilities

- facial features, feeding difficulties, small stature

- psychiatric disorder

Syndrome Definition . . . .

Velocardiofacial syndrome (VCFS) is a relatively common genetic condition with over 170 known traits (Gerber, 1998). The original phenotype was described in 1967 by Sedlockova, and Dr. Robert J. Shprintzen is credited with further delineating this condition from others in 1978. It is the most common syndrome associated with a cleft palate, occurring in approximately five to eight percent of children born with a cleft palate (NIDOCD, 1996).

Velocardiofacial syndrome has an autosomal dominant pattern of heredity. Those affected have a 50% chance of having a child with this syndrome, but only 10-15% of cases have it as an inherited trait. The specific chromosomal deletion responsible for Velocardiofacial syndrome is found on chromosome 22 and is considered a microdeletion based on its size (Batshaw, 1997). VCFS is reported in 1/700 live births.

Features vary among children, but the most common ones include heart defects, cleft palate (usually the velum), learning problems, feeding difficulties, and speech disorders.

Specific facial features include an elongated face, and a wide, long, tubular nose with a prominent root and a dimpled tip. Small ears are noted, with attached lobules and unfurled helices. Almond-shaped eyes with puffy upper eyelids can appear narrow and slit-like due to the narrowness of the palpebral fissures. A down-turned oral commissure and small mouth are seen, and the face is "masklike" (Gerber, 1998). A mild facial asymmetry, flattened malar eminences, micrognathia, and retrognathia have also been reported. At least 15% of patients with Pierre Robin sequence have Velocardiofacial syndrome.

Velocardiofacial Syndrome is also known as:

- Shprintzen Syndrome
- Craniofacial Syndrome
- Conotruncal Anomaly Unusual Face Syndrome
- Deletion #22q11.2 Syndrome

Some of the specific heart defects associated with VCFS include ventral septal defects, right-sided aortic arch defects, and tetralogy of Fallot. Other cardial defects range from mild to profound, depending on the child.

Velocardiofacial syndrome is often undiagnosed because many of the characteristics can be minor and frequently occur in the general population. The facial feature profile may be the most consistent diagnostic factor for Velocardiofacial syndrome. Congenital heart defects may be seen but there is wide variance as to the severity.

An MRI can detect soft tissue anomalies, and children with Velocardiofacial syndrome typically have cysts near the ventricles (Shprintzen, 1997). Other medical symptoms include kidney and vascular anomalies, visual

---

The syndrome name contains the three most affected structures/systems.

Velo	=	velum, or soft palate
Cardio	=	heart
Facial	=	face

---

deformities, and immune system abnormalities. A mild growth deficiency with scoliosis and small hands may also be observed.

The behavioral characteristics associated with Velocardiofacial syndrome are explained in the following section.

Infant Feeding Problems

Infant feeding difficulties are correlated with Velocardiofacial syndrome. Pharyngeal hypotonicity, found in 90% of the population, will interfere with accurate feeding movements. A weak sucking pattern, nasal regurgitation, and gastroesophageal reflux are all reported. Upper airway obstruction and Pierre Robin sequence are common in these infants and will affect feeding movements. The child might also fail to thrive.

Learning Disabilities

Learning disabilities are part of all known cases of Velocardiofacial syndrome (Gerber, 1998). Early testing in the cognitive area may be within normal limits but as children enter school, their cognitive deficits will probably increase. Reading comprehension and mathematical reasoning are specific areas of difficulty, possibly due to the high level of abstraction for optimal performance. Rote counting and basic reading skills will be intact and attention deficit hyperactivity disorder is also observed.

Mental Retardation

Children with VCFS appear to have intellectual functioning within normal limits until about age 6. At that point, they continue to function at a concrete cognitive level with poor abstracting abilities. These concrete learning patterns will probably last throughout life. A mild mental retardation is reported in 40% of these children (Gerber, 1998), and many others will not be eligible for special education services because they will test in the lowest range of typical intellectual functioning. The recurrent, fluctuating hearing loss found with otitis media will put these children at further risk academically.

Mental Illness

Some adolescents and adults with Velocardiofacial syndrome will develop attention deficit hyperactivity disorders (ADHD), depression, bipolar disorder, and generalized anxiety. Paranoid schizophrenia, obsessive compulsive disorders, and severe personality disorders are evidenced. The psychiatric disorders were recognized as part of this syndrome in 1992 (Sphrintzen, 1997).

Speech-Language Issues . . . .

You should be aware of several specific aspects of the communication profile in VCFS.

Voice Disorders

Voice disorders are very common in children with VCFS. Hypernasality is common, may involve nasal emissions, and is often severe. Causes for the hypernasality include cleft palate, short velum, deep pharyngeal cavity, palatal weakness or incoordination, and lateral wall dysfunction or pharyngeal hypotonia. Other voice and resonance characteristics are hoarseness, cul-de-sac resonance patterns, and reduced intraoral breath pressure or denasality. Hypernasality can be masked by hoarseness and should be evaluated very carefully.

Hearing Concerns

Hearing loss is common in children with Velocardiofacial syndrome. The majority of these losses are conductive and are secondary to otitis media. Recurrent ear infections and upper respiratory infections secondary to a compromised immune system are both seen in VCFS, as are ossicular chain malformations. Sensorineural losses are seen in 15% of the population (Shprintzen, 1997).

Speech/Phonological Disorders

Speech development may be delayed due to a number of factors. Structural defects such as cleft palate, micrognathia, and hypotonicity will affect feeding movements and prespeech movements. Dental anomalies such as enamel hypoplasia and congenitally missing teeth will affect phoneme production. Children with VCFS typically don't develop pharyngeal fricatives, pharyngeal stops, and mid-dorsal stops, and will use global glottal stop substitutes, particularly in cases with cleft or velopharyngeal insufficiency. This compensatory articulatory pattern is well-documented. Phonological delays or disorders, dyspraxia, and dysarthria may also be seen.

Language Impairment

Language development is delayed and language disorders are common. These children appear to display intellectual and language functioning within normal limits until about age 6, when they do not move from a concrete level of cognition. Advanced mental representation and abstraction abilities will not develop as the children age. Specific deficits in auditory memory and processing are noted (Shprintzen, 1997).

Intervention Issues

- Early Intervention

- Special Education

- Voice Disorders

- Speech/Phonological Therapy

- Language Therapy

- Team Approach

Intervention Issues . . . .

Here are some things to keep in mind when considering intervention for clients with VCFS.

Early Intervention

- Perform an early, accurate diagnosis for children to ensure that they will receive the earliest intervention possible.

- Use a team approach in early intervention with an emphasis on cognition, language, and communication.

- Provide early attention to feeding structures and nutrition input.

Special Education

- Due to the relationship between learning disabilities and mental retardation in Velocardiofacial syndrome, special education and related services for school-aged children should be in place.

- Provide intensive work in the content areas of mathematics and reading because these have been singled out as curricular deficit areas.

- Clients with VCFS will probably have life-long cognitive challenges, especially in abstract thinking.

- A poor prognosis for complete habilation has been reported.

Voice Disorders

- Complete evaluations of the oral and nasal structures and the pharynges prior to treatment. Nasopharyngoscopy may reveal the cause of any exhibited hypernasality. The child may need surgery that includes cleft closure or a pharyngeal flap procedure. There are complications with each of these surgical choices, including cardiac involvement and abnormal blood vessels, which affect the outcome.

- Use a prosthetic device if you can treat the velopharyngeal insufficiency without surgery or if surgery is going to be delayed pending more tissue growth.

- Children with VCFS have a high incidence of recurrent ear infections with upper respiratory infections. A child who is undiagnosed might be a candidate for an adenoidectomy, but this surgery in combination with an undetected submucous cleft can result in postsurgical velopharyngeal insufficiency. Provide early, accurate diagnosis.

Speech/Phonological Therapy

- Traditional articulation therapy with behavior management strategies may work for specific phonemic errors. Practice difficult consonants with the client (including fricatives and stops), particularly those made near the pharyngeal area.

- Eliminating the frequency of glottal stop substitutions will greatly improve overall intelligibility.

- If an assessment of speech production suggests a phonological disorder, conduct two deeper types of analysis. Take a phonemic inventory; note the production of the number and variety of consonants and vowels; and compare them to age norms. You can also take a relational inventory which could include examining the child's production as compared to adult productions. The goal is to increase the number of phonemes in a child's repertoire and increase frequency of use.

Language Therapy

- Provide early language stimulation because children with VCFS have a tendency to plateau in their language development in early childhood.

- School-aged children will need language therapy to assist with abstract thinking, auditory memory, and auditory processing skills.

- Language abilities may parallel cognitive abilities, and if children are in the range of mental retardation, initiate language for life span planning.

- People with VCFS can develop mental illnesses in adolescence and adulthood; therefore, develop language therapies that are reality-oriented.

Team Approach

- In addition to the professions mentioned above, medical professionals should also be team members because the syndrome presents such a complicated medical profile, with indications of abnormalities in many of the body's systems.

- If available, a craniofacial or cleft palate team can provide appropriate treatment. Audiologists; prosthedontists; surgeons; and ear, nose and throat doctors can also contribute.

- Include family members in any team providing treatment for children with VCFS. The inclusion of families as team members assists in smooth transition from early intervention to school-based services.

- In later years, psychiatric and mental health professionals should be involved to manage the symptoms of VCFS.

Summary ·

Velocardiofacial syndrome is a relatively common genetic condition with an autosomal dominant pattern of heredity. The most commonly found features include heart defects, cleft palate (usually the velum), characteristic facial features, learning problems, feeding difficulties, and speech disorders. VCFS often goes undiagnosed because many characteristics can be minor and may be found in the general population. There is variance as to which features will be found in each child.

There are many specific speech-language difficulties. Voice disorders (particularly hypernasality and velopharyngeal insufficiency) are most common. Surgical, prosthetic, and therapeutic management from a team perspective are recommended for voice issues. Speech disorders may result from structural deficiencies. The client might also exhibit phonological disorders, dyspraxia, and dysarthria.

Intellectual functioning and language development are areas of concern in this population. Children can develop cognitively within normal limits until age 6, then they have marked inabilities to think abstractly. This concrete learning style continues throughout life and tends to hurt the child academically. Special education is generally necessary if the child is eligible. Many children will not test in this range, and therefore might not receive special education services. A team approach is best for treatment of VCFS from both a medical and an educational perspective.

References

Batshaw, M. L. *Children with Disabilities, Fourth Edition.* Baltimore, MD: Paul H. Brookes Publishing Co., 1997.

Batshaw, M. & Perret, Y. *Children with Disabilities—A Medical Primer, Third Edition.* Baltimore, MD: Paul H. Brookes Publishing Co., 1992.

Carneol, S. O. & Marks, S. M. "The Speech-Language Pathologist: Key Role in the Diagnosis of Velocardiofacial Syndrome." *American Journal of Speech-Language Pathology*, 8, pp. 23-32, 1999.

Gerber, S. E. *Etiology and Prevention of Communicative Disorders, Second Edition.* San Diego, CA: Singular Publishing Group, Inc., 1998.

"Information on Velocardiofacial Syndrome." National Institutes on Deafness and Other Communication Disorders. Bethesda, MD: NIDCD Information Clearinghouse, 1996.

McWilliams, B. J., Moris, H. L., & Shelton, R. L. *Cleft Palate Speech, Second Edition.* Philadelphia, PA: B.C. Decker, Inc., 1990.

Shprintzen, R. J. *Genetics, Syndromes, and Communication Disorders.* San Diego, CA: Singular Publishing Group, Inc., 1997.

Shprintzen, R. J. & Bardach, J. *Cleft Palate Speech Management: A Multi-disciplinary Approach.* St. Louis, MO: Mosby Year Book, 1995.

Notes

Waardenburg Syndrome

Characteristics

- Hearing impairment
- Vision impairment
- Speech-language delays

- unusual eye shape

- eyes of different colors

- white forelock

- small nose

- deafness/hearing impairment

- 1/20,000-40,000 live births

Syndrome Definition . . . .

Children with Waardenburg syndrome have striking, unusual facial anomalies, but the impact of the disorder is usually minimal beyond appearance. The head and neck area are usually the primary affected features. There are also differences in hair and skin pigmentation, eyes, nose, and eyebrows. Other affected features can be deafness, glaucoma, depigmented areas of skin, and clefts of the lip and/or palate in rare cases.

Waardenburg syndrome is an inherited, autosomal-dominant condition, probably located on chromosome 9. Incidence is reported in the range of one in every 20,000 to one in every 40,000 live births. Males and females are equally affected. There are three distinct subtypes of the syndrome, and they are defined by the presence and severity of the specific characteristics. All characteristics of the syndrome are confined to the head and neck region, with the exception of subtype 3, which includes abnormalities in the upper limbs. The limb anomalies may include lack of arm growth, extra fingers, fused fingers, or finger malformations.

Almost all children with Waardenburg exhibit an unusual eye shape. The inner edges of the eyes tend to be farther away from the usual midline position against the bridge of the nose. This position can affect the opening of the lower tear ducts, causing some problems in the flow of tears. Perhaps one of the more striking features of the eyes is the difference in color between the two. For example, one eye might be light blue while the other is dark brown. While the deviant coloring of the iris does not compromise vision, glaucoma can begin. Glaucoma is a dangerous increase in tension inside the eyeball which is measured by elevated pressures. Children with Waardenburg syndrome may be more susceptible to glaucoma because of the unusual structure of the orbit of the eyeball, making normal drainage somewhat difficult.

Another unusual feature is the eyebrow line. The eyebrows tend to grow across the forehead until they meet in the middle over the upper bridge of the nose. Not everyone showing this eyebrow pattern has Waardenburg, but it can help make a definitive diagnosis. Children tend to have small noses that remain proportionately small on their faces throughout life. This can cause frequent blockage, leading to chronic upper-respiratory infections. These children tend to be mouth breathers as a result of small nasal passages.

It's typical for the child with Waardenburg to exhibit a completely white fore-lock on the forehead, which can be present at birth even with a dark head of hair. Occasionally, the white forelock will fade or disappear in childhood but reappear during adolescence. Head and all facial hair is also prone to premature greying, sometimes by as early as 17-20 years of age.

Deafness is the most serious feature, affecting approximately 25% of those with the disorder. The sensorineural hearing loss can be unilateral (one ear) or bilateral (both ears). It is critical that a severe hearing loss be diagnosed early so that speech-language services can be implemented and other aspects of normal development not be significantly compromised. Development of voice and language generally proceed normally unless they're impaired secondarily by the hearing loss. Approximately 5% of cases also have clefts of the lip and/or palate. Depending on severity and success of surgical intervention, you may need to introduce compensatory articulation positions in speech-language therapy.

Behavioral Characteristics Profile . . . .

The behavioral characteristics associated with Waardenburg syndrome are explained in the following section.

Hearing Impairment

One prominent feature is congenital sensorineural hearing impairment. The degree of hearing loss ranges from mild to severe, and can be

Speech-Language Issues

• Hearing

• Articulation

• Resonance

• Language

unilateral or bilateral. If the child is profoundly deaf, early speech-language intervention will be critical for development of communication skills. Special education services may also be necessary later if the deafness is profound and bilateral. Lesser degrees of hearing loss will have a minimal impact on academic and communication progress.

Hearing acuity should be monitored regularly throughout early childhood. Parents should be alerted to watch for difficulties that a child might demonstrate at home. Routine checks should pick up hearing loss if it's not detected during newborn screening procedures.

Vision Impairment

Visual acuity is not affected by the different colors of the eyes. However, glaucoma can occur. Parents and teachers should be alerted to any reports of pain in the child's eyes, blurred vision, and halos around lights. Eyedrops or surgery may be necessary if high pressure is present in the eyes.

Speech-Language Delays

Delays in acquisition of speech and language skills will be secondary to the primary impairments of hearing and cleft palate. If these features are not present in the Waardenburg profile, then speech-language development should proceed normally. The severity of hearing and cleft features will directly influence the degree of difficulty the individual might experience in acquiring communication skills and subsequent academic progress.

Speech-Language Issues . . . .

Speech-language issues in Waardenburg syndrome are caused by the severe sensorineural hearing impairment from birth. Newborn/infant screening programs can have a critical impact on diagnosis. The sooner hearing loss is detected and diagnosed, the better the long-term prognosis. Professionals can begin focusing intervention efforts on the aspects of speech-language development that are likely to be affected by the hearing impairment.

The other aspect that can affect speech production is the presence of a cleft lip and/or palate. Surgical intervention or prosthesis may resolve many of the issues, but motor movement patterns for sound production and resonance balance will probably have to be addressed.

Hearing

Congenital deafness is often a symptom of the disorder. The organ of Corti may be absent in some children. Most hearing losses are static and present at birth, but in Type 2, the hearing loss can be progressive. The severity of the loss will directly affect the degree of speech-language impairments. Amplification and visual stimulation can be considered to compensate for the impaired auditory channel.

Articulation

Production of sounds for expressive communication can be significantly impacted by the loss of hearing. Hearing aids might compensate to allow an auditory model for some sounds, but oral-motor postures should be introduced with visual aids to teach speech production. Compensatory movements may be necessary if clefts of the lip and/or palate compromise movement patterns.

Resonance

Voice production is usually within normal parameters, but resonance balance can be impaired by the hearing loss. Hypernasality can be a problem if cleft palate is present as part of the syndrome.

Language

Language development will be affected secondarily by the hearing loss. Early intervention can insure a solid language foundation to prevent later academic deficits when language stimulation is initiated as soon as problems become apparent.

Intervention issues with Waardenburg syndrome deal strongly with a team approach. Here is a summary.

Intervention Issues

- Hearing

- Speech Production

- Language

- Team Approach

Hearing

- If the child is a candidate for amplification, have an audiologist select appropriate hearing aids for sensori-neural loss.

- Communication input should be consistent with the degree of hearing impairment regarding use of sign language or other deaf education techniques.

Speech Production

- Teach oral-motor postures using visual and tactile stimulation to compensate for hearing deficits.

- Compensatory positions may be necessary if structural deviations are present due to cleft lip and/or palate.

- Implement exercises to strengthen velopharyngeal closure if hypernasality or resonance deviations are present due to cleft.

Language

- Receptive and expressive language acquisition will be critical to general development. Language forms the foundation for academic learning and prognosis will be significantly impacted by whether comprehension and expression of communication can be established.

- Use language techniques consistent with principles of deaf education (i.e., stimulating through multisensory modality) at an early age to develop an awareness of semantic meanings through concrete experiences.

Team Approach

- An audiologist should conduct periodic evaluations to monitor the child's hearing loss (particularly if it becomes worse) and assess possible benefits from amplification or other technology.

- An ophthamologist should do periodic checks on eye pressures to monitor for the possible onset of glaucoma.

- A teacher trained in deaf education might be necessary to consult on educational placement and strategies to promote learning in the school setting.

Summary . . . .

Children with Waardenburg syndrome have rather striking facial appearances which include irises of different colors, a white forelock of hair, a small nose, and eyebrows that grow together across the forehead at the upper bridge of the nose. Congenital deafness or some degree of sensorineural hearing loss can be present in one or both ears. Possible additional characteristics can include glaucoma, cleft lip and/or palate, lack of pigmentation in areas of the skin, widely-spaced eyes, and occasional limb anomalies. Children tend to grey prematurely in facial and head hair (sometimes as early as 17-20 years of age). Milder cases of the syndrome are not always recognized until a more severely affected member of the family has been diagnosed with Waardenburg syndrome, and physical deviations in other family members are subsequently analyzed.

Future prognosis depends on the presence and severity of hearing problems. If hearing is normal, the physical features should not affect the client's ability to learn, future career choices, and future leisure activities. The only feature with potential life-long implications is the hearing loss and subsequent acquisition of a communication system. The early initiation of speech-language services to establish a communication foundation and prevent academic problems can offer a normal prognosis for people with Waardenburg.

References

Batshaw, M. & Perret, Y. *Children with Disabilities—A Medical Primer, Third Edition.* Baltimore, MD: Paul H. Brookes Publishing Co., 1992.

Gilbert, P. *The A-Z Reference Book of Syndromes and Inherited Disorders, Second Edition.* New York, NY: Chapman & Hall, 1996.

Shprintzen, R. J. *Genetics, Syndromes, and Communication Disorders.* San Diego, CA: Singular Publishing Group, Inc., 1997.

Notes . . . .

Conclusion

"How silent the woods would be if only the best birds sang."

Anonymous

This quote appears in a delightful little book called *Love Adds a Little Chocolate* by Medard Laz. It serves as a reminder of why we struggle to develop speech-language skills in young children who already have the odds stacked against them. Children diagnosed early in life with a syndrome disability will probably never achieve perfection or "normal" communication skills. Their physical structures and/or neurology are genetically wired in a different way that prevents realistic achievement of that goal. But functional skills are not unattainable. The level of competence might be low on a continuum of ability, but small steps are monumental achievements for some of these exceptional children.

Variety and differences contribute to keeping the world interesting. If everyone looked the same, had the same talents, and demonstrated identical skills, the joy of new discoveries would be lost. Creative innovations are often bred by necessity. When "normal" doesn't work, something different must be tried. Those who march to a different drummer need to be encouraged to march, not be discouraged from even trying because they can't march like the majority. Children with syndrome disabilities add challenges, insights, and opportunities for the rest of us. They need to be encouraged and assisted in their efforts to join in the song of life.

We continue to be amazed and humbled by the neuroplasticity of the brain to compensate and recover limited skills when intervention efforts are initiated early in life. Research continues to demonstrate dramatic improvement in speech-language ability when remediation efforts begin as soon as possible.

Medical technology also continues to demonstrate tremendous improvements in repairing compromised physical and neurological structures. Genetic research creeps closer and closer to discovering the cause of various disabilities through chromosome mapping. Tissue transplants and generation offer promising hopes for regrowing deficit structures. The new century is pulsating with exciting possibilities in medical research. The syndrome descriptions and prognoses of the past are no longer true, and the future descriptions may be very different from the present. Professionals must balance the syndrome's present reality with the hopes of a brighter future.

Families prepare for the birth of new child with great hope and dreams for the future. When diagnosed with a syndrome at birth or shortly after, many parents speak of it as feeling like the breath was knocked from their bodies.

They can scarcely breathe or think as their hopes and dreams are crushed under the weight of a syndrome label.

Speech-language pathologists are often the first professionals to become involved in regular remediation sessions with the family and child. We have the opportunity to slowly piece together some of those shattered dreams. The road to improvement may be long, tedious, painful, time-consuming, frustrating, expensive, and scary. It's difficult to keep trudging down that path if no hope is offered for the end. The realities are ever-present and someone needs to provide a glimpse beyond the current struggle toward progress and a measure of success. A story from one of the parents we have worked with illustrates this idea quite well.

The family's first child, a daughter, was not developing as expected. The parents took the eighteen-month-old to a major medical clinical for diagnosis. A syndrome label was introduced as well as dire predictions for the future. The young mother and father were told that their daughter was profoundly mentally retarded and would never function independently. She would never talk, feed herself, dress herself, be toilet trained, etc. The parents were advised to put the girl in an institution and get on with their lives.

> If everyone looked the same, had the same talents, and demonstrated identical skills, the joy of new discoveries would be lost.

The parents could not accept the recommendation. They decided that this was their daughter, their flesh and blood. If she had significant problems, so be it. But she was a member of their family and would grow up being loved and cared for in their home.

The mother began educating herself on the disability and pursuing therapeutic services to stimulate development in her daughter. Speech-language therapists, occupational therapists, physical therapists, and special education professionals were hired and trained to implement techniques in the home. The daughter began responding over time and the parents were encouraged by the progress reports and impressions shared by the intervention professionals. Stimulation, love, support, and perseverance were paying off. The professionals were giving the parents hope that maybe the dire predictions of the future were not accurate. Verbal language started to emerge and motor skills started to develop. A younger sister born in the family provided a developmental model for the older daughter to keep pace with and to imitate.

There were lots of tears, lots of frustration, and lots of embarrassment in public situations. The mother is the first to tell you that there were days she wanted to give it all up. But hope for the future and the increasing quality of her daughter's life kept them all going. Speech-language pathologists saw different things in the behavior and interaction of the little girl over time that negated some of the conclusions introduced at eighteen months to the family.

The end result was, and continues to be, an inspiring story. The little girl started kindergarten in regular education with chronologically age-appropriate peers. Supplemental services the first year included a one-on-one aide, speech-language therapy, and occupational therapy. Intensity of services faded over time and by second grade, the girl was a verbal chatterbox. She completed academic work with her peers, took care of her own needs, and even showed me a bandage on her knee from a fall when she'd been riding her bike. She's now doing fine in school with minimal learning disabilities assistance and speech-language therapy services.

She's not perfect. She's still different from her peers in some ways. The mother made some enemies along the way with her demands and expectations for her daughter. The family definitely experienced peaks and valleys. The destination has not been reached, and unique challenges will continue to present themselves over time.

We don't have a crystal ball to predict the future. As SLPs, we have a responsibility to introduce present descriptions of deficits and recommend intervention goals, but it's not within our expertise to say where the child might be as an adult. The future reality is not a constant; it changes rapidly. We have to begin our therapy services at the present level of a child's abilities, and allow the future to unfold in its own time—and with hope!

"What oxygen is to the lungs, such is hope to the meaning of life."
Emil Brunner

●   ●   ●   ●   ●   ●   ●

	Apert	Beckwith-Wiedemann	CHARGE	Cri-du-Chat	Crouzon	Goldenhar	Klinefelter
Age of Onset	birth	birth	birth	birth	birth	birth	birth
Cause	chromosome 10	varies	chromosome 22	chromosome 5	chromosome 10	unknown	extra X chromosome
Incidence	1/100,000-160,000	7/10,000	1/12,000	1/20,000-50,000	unknown	1/5,600-45,000	1/500-1000 (men)
Syndrome Deficits							
Cognitive/Mental	x	x	x	x	x		x
Cleft Lip/Palate	x	x	x	x		x	
Stature		x	x	x			
Motor		x		x			x
Physical/Facial	x	x	x	x	x	x	
Seizures							
Vision			x		x	x	
Hearing	x		x		x	x	
Other Health Issues	x	x	x	x			
Speech-Language Issues							
Auditory/Hearing	x		x			x	
Feeding/Swallowing	x			x		x	
Language	x	x	x	x	x	x	x
Resonance/Voice	x	x	x	x	x	x	
Articulation	x	x	x	x	x	x	x
Intervention							
Special Education	x		x	x	x		x
PT/OT		x		x		x	
Audiologist	x		x	x	x	x	x
Ophthamologist			x		x	x	
Orthodontist	x	x			x	x	
Surgical/Medical	x	x	x	x	x	x	x

	Sotos	Cornelia de Lange	Moebius	MPS	Noonan	Pierre Robin
Age of Onset	birth	birth	birth	birth	birth	birth
Cause	chromosome 3	chromosome 3 or 17	mutation	varies	genetic	birth defect
Incidence	very rare	1/50,000	rare	1/16,000-216,000	1/1,000-2,500	1/2,000-1/30,000
Syndrome Deficits						
Cognitive/Mental	x	x		x	x	x
Cleft Lip/Palate		x			x	x
Stature	x	x		x	x	
Motor	x	x	x	x	x	
Physical/Facial	x	x	x	x	x	x
Seizures		x				
Vision		x		x	x	
Hearing		x		x	x	x
Other Health Issues	x	x		x	x	x
Speech-Language Issues						
Auditory/Hearing		x		x	x	x
Feeding/Swallowing	x	x	x		x	x
Language	x	x	x	x	x	x
Resonance/Voice		x	x		x	x
Articulation	x	x	x		x	x
Intervention						
Special Education		x		x	x	x
PT/OT		x	x	x	x	x
Audiologist		x			x	x
Ophthamologist			x	x	x	
Orthodontist					x	x
Surgical/Medical	x	x	x	x	x	x

	Stickler	Sturge-Weber	Treacher Collins	Usher	VCFS	Waarden-burg
Age of Onset	birth	birth	birth	birth	birth	birth
Cause	chromosome 12 and 6	mutation	chromosome 5	genetic	chromosome 22	chromosome 9
Incidence	1/10,000	rare	1/10,000-50,000	3/5,000-10,000	1/700	1/20,000 40,000
Syndrome Deficits						
Cognitive/Mental		x		x	x	
Cleft Lip/Palate	x				x	x
Stature						
Motor	x	x		x		
Physical/Facial	x	x	x		x	x
Seizures		x				
Vision	x	x		x		x
Hearing	x		x	x	x	x
Other Health Issues	x				x	
Speech-Language Issues						
Auditory/Hearing	x		x	x	x	x
Feeding/Swallowing	x		x		x	
Language		x		x	x	x
Resonance/Voice	x	x	x	x	x	x
Articulation	x	x	x	x	x	x
Intervention						
Special Education		x		x	x	x
PT/OT		x				
Audiologist	x		x	x	x	x
Ophthamologist	x	x		x		x
Orthodontist	x	x	x			
Surgical/Medical	x	x	x		x	

19-03-98765